The Truth about the Aids Panic

Dr Michael Fitzpatrick
Don Milligan

junius

Fitzpatrick, Dr Michael and Milligan, Don

The Truth about the Aids Panic
1. Medical Science
2. Politics
3. Sociology

I Title
ISBN 0 948392 07 X

Published March 1987
Typeset by Junius Publications Ltd (TU)
Printed by Russell Press (TU)

Contents

Preface

We had long been aware of the climate of public prejudice about Aids that was being whipped up by the tabloid press. But it was not until November last year, when the government officially sponsored the Aids scare, that we really began to take notice.

One of us, working as a GP, was appalled at the distress caused to people who had not the slightest risk of contracting Aids. Elderly men worried about some sexual misdemeanour 30 years ago, anxious parents terrified about the dangers to their children in school changing rooms and public swimming baths, women working alongside gay men—all came rushing in for advice and reassurance. While the Aids obsession swept the media, including the medical press, real health problems were neglected.

The other, after more than a decade of active involvement in the cause of gay liberation, was shocked at the way the gay movement had been dragged on to the 'safe sex' bandwagon alongside Tory politicians and right-wing moralists. The British left too appeared to take the government's campaign against Aids at face value and restricted its response to demanding more of the same.

Before Christmas we got together to write an account of Aids that would try to cut through the prejudice that surrounds it and clarify what were the real issues at stake. This pamphlet is the result.

The first part examines the evidence about the spread of Aids. In particular it critically assesses the validity of the government's claim that it is a serious risk to heterosexuals in Britain. For those who want to know more about the virus and how it works, we have presented a brief survey of the current state of knowledge. We also outline the anatomy of a moral panic and the consequences of such irrational movements, particularly at a time of wider social instability. We argue that Aids is not a problem for most people, and that its spread among gay men can only be tackled by ending discrimination against homosexuality.

In the second part of the pamphlet, we look at the convergence of the government, the professional moralists, the medical profession and the gay movement around the safe sex campaign. We examine in particular the impact of Aids on the gay movement in the USA and in Britain, and the way in which the left too has gone along with the Aids panic. In conclusion, we look at the importance of Victorian family values to the British establishment and the dangers of the drive to enforce them on the rest of society.

We do not regard the Aids scare as a conspiracy, but as something much more insidious. It reflects the concern of a threatened establishment to strengthen its grip over society by seizing any opportunity to promote the values of conformity and discipline. The success of the government in winning such a wide range of support for its campaign, and in creating a climate of fear affecting millions, shows the weakness of the official forces of opposition on this as on so many issues. In what is likely to be an election year, we cannot afford to let an offensive which carries such profound consequences go unchallenged.

Michael Fitzpatrick
Don Milligan
London,
February 1987

Anybody who would like to get involved in campaigning against the Aids scare can contact us by writing to Junius Publications, BCM JPLtd, London WC1N 3XX, or by phoning (01) 729 3771.

1. 'Why should you be concerned about Aids?'

'Why be concerned?' asks 'Aids: Don't Die of Ignorance', the special leaflet the government had delivered to 23 million British households in January. Here is the official answer:

> 'Any man or woman can get the Aids virus depending on their behaviour. It is not just a homosexual disease.
> 'There is no cure. And it kills.
> 'By the time you read this, probably 300 people will have died in this country. It is believed that a further 30 000 carry the virus. This number is rising and will continue to rise unless we all take precautions.'

The clipped prose sounds convincing, but is the message accurate? Will Aids really spread unchecked 'unless we all take precautions'? First, let's look at how Aids spreads.

The Aids virus has been found in a wide range of body fluids—saliva, tears,.breast milk and vaginal secretions. But only blood and semen act as effective *transmitters* of the infection. It appears, however, that the virus can also pass from a pregnant woman to the baby in her womb.

How you can't catch Aids

The Aids virus cannot be passed on by ordinary social contact, by coughing and sneezing, hugging and kissing, or by the shared use of washing and cooking utensils or of toilet facilities. Numerous exposures of parents, siblings and others to the various body fluids of children who have contracted Aids have resulted in the transmission of the virus in not a single case. Many accidental exposures of laboratory staff—even many needle-stick injuries—have failed to lead to infection. One nurse in Britain who accidentally injected herself with a small quantity of contaminated blood has become infected with the Aids virus, but that is the only known case in the Western world.

There has been some controversy over a case in which a woman was presumed to have become infected via her husband's saliva, and another in which a child was thought to have been infected by a bite on the forearm from his brother (*The Lancet,* 22/29 December 1984 and 20 September 1986). But Donald Acheson, the government's chief medical adviser, echoes all expert thinking with his conclusion that 'There is no sound evidence that the virus has been transmitted by kissing' (*Guardian,* 30 January 1987).

Medical officialdom has designated the Aids virus a relatively low risk to everybody caring for Aids patients or examining their body fluids. Only routine precautions are required (see Advisory Committee on Dangerous Pathogens, 'LAV/HTLV III: The Causative Agent of Aids and Related Conditions', Revised guidelines, June 1986).

The low infectiousness of the Aids virus did not deter a Metropolitan Police squad from donning rubber gloves when they raided a gay bar in Vauxhall, London in January 1987. Nor did it stop Dr John O'Hara, a 79-year old GP from Rottingdean, Sussex, from advising the Football Association to recommend that footballers stop sharing post-match baths and bottles of champagne. O'Hara did point out that there was no harm in players 'dry-kissing on the cheek', but noted that the FA 'disapproved of the habit'. The Aids virus is not very infectious—but the government leaflet goes to some lengths to avoid clarifying this point.

How you can catch Aids

There is no doubt that the Aids virus can be transmitted through blood. There have been many cases of Aids among haemophiliacs, who require periodic transfusions of blood products. Others who have received blood transfusions, following accidents or operations, have also caught the virus in this way. Again, drug addicts who share needles and syringes with other addicts have contracted Aids.

There is also strong evidence that the Aids virus can be transmitted in semen. A high proportion of Aids cases in the West are homosexual men. It appears that anal intercourse is associated with a high risk of transmitting the virus. It seems that semen containing the virus can

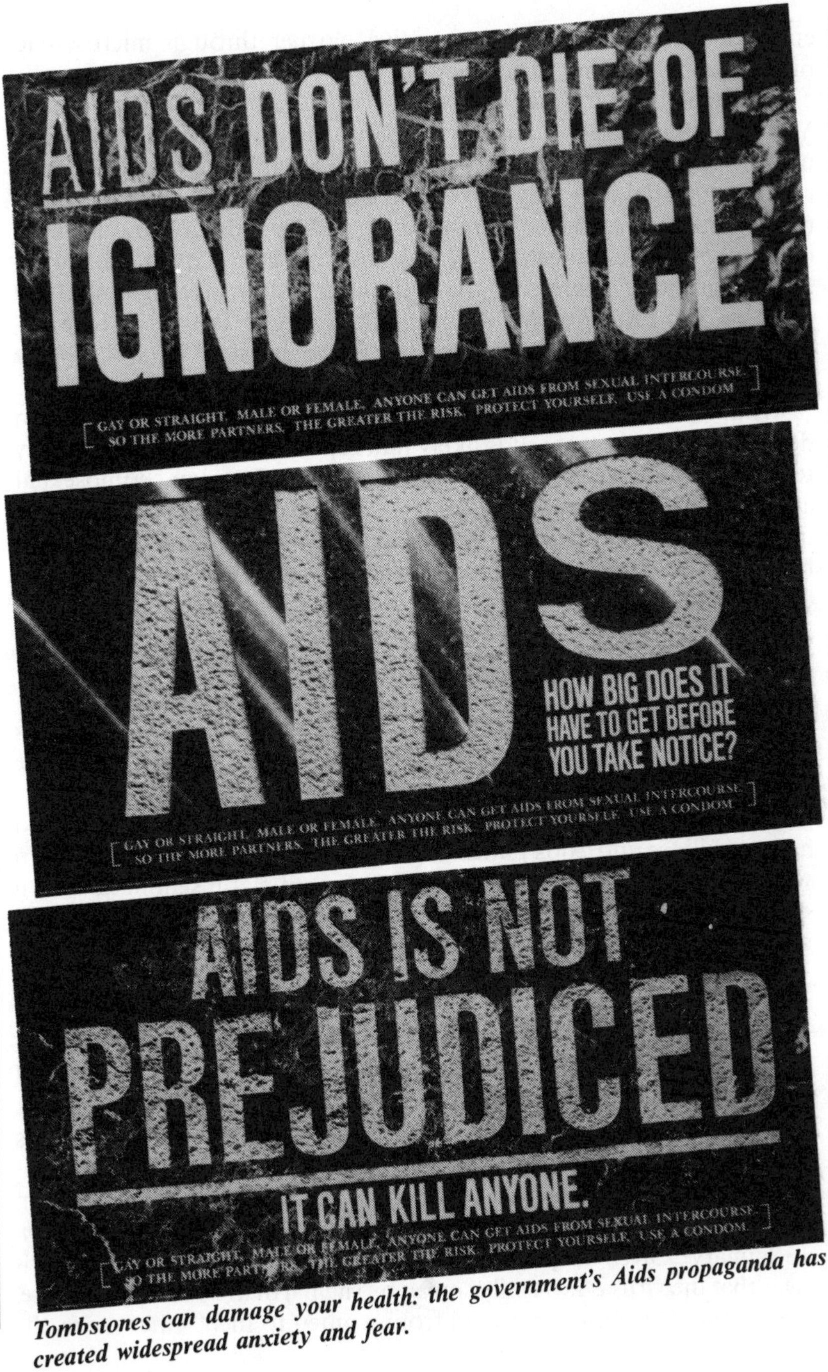

Tombstones can damage your health: the government's Aids propaganda has created widespread anxiety and fear.

enter the circulation of the receptive partner through microscopic breaches in the lining of his rectum.

A team led by Dr Brian Evans, head of genitourinary medicine at the West London hospital, recently made a study of more than 300 gay men in London (*Genitourinary Medicine,* December 1986). The team's report concludes that only the receptive partner in anal intercourse is at risk. It found no evidence of transmission of the Aids virus by oral-anal or oral-genital contact, or by swallowing semen. A much larger American survey confirms these findings. After investigating 1000 men, the San Francisco Men's Health Study argues that receptive anal-genital contact is 'the major mode of transmission' (*Journal of the American Medical Association,* 16 January 1987).

What transmits the Aids virus among gay men is infected semen deposited in the rectum. It is likely that repeated exposure is necessary to transmit the virus: in the Evans survey in London, homosexual activity for more than five years was the strongest predictor of infection. Likewise, the San Francisco study noted a clear association between the number of male sexual partners and the likelihood of infection.

What about heterosexuals?

The question of the heterosexual transmission of the Aids virus is contentious. There is some evidence that infected men can pass the virus to their female sexual partners by vaginal intercourse. Antibodies to the Aids virus have been observed in the partners of infected haemophiliacs and Aids patients. There have also been a few cases in which women became infected following artificial insemination with semen from a carrier of the Aids virus. Again semen seems to be the key factor in transmission.

While it is *possible* for the Aids virus to be passed from men to women in vaginal intercourse, in the West relatively few women appear to have been infected in this way. By the end of 1986, only 10 British women were thought to have acquired Aids from men by the vaginal route, and only three of these actually caught the infection in this country. In the USA, by the end of 1985, 151 women had acquired Aids through heterosexual contact, at a time when the total of cases stood at more than 18 000. Heterosexual anal intercourse may be a factor in some of these cases (see *Journal of the American Medical Association,* 16 January). Given the prevalence of bisexuality among gay men, it seems clear that the virus is less easily spread by vaginal than by anal intercourse.

Can the Aids virus be passed from women to men? Once more, the

Aids virus has been *found* in both cervical and vaginal secretions, but uncertainty still surrounds whether it can be effectively *transmitted* by this route. One American survey which purports to demonstrate the infection of servicemen by contact with prostitutes has been criticised on methodological grounds (see *Journal of the American Medical Association,* 18 October 1985 and 4 April 1986).

Up to the end of 1986 there were but 10 cases of men in Britain who had apparently acquired Aids through heterosexual contact. Only one of these cases, it seems, actually picked up the infection in Britain. In the USA, up to the end of 1985, some 28 men were considered to have been infected by heterosexual contact—0.2 per cent of the total number of male Aids sufferers. Sexual contact with female drug users was a factor in most of these cases (see *The Lancet,* 22 March 1986).

The main evidence for the spread of the Aids virus from women to men comes from studies in Africa which show similar levels of infection among men and women. Some experts postulate a central role for prostitutes in transmitting the infection in Africa (for a recent survey, see *British Medical Journal,* 6 December 1986). But this case is far from proven. As a result of the prevalence of malnutrition and chronic parasitic infection in Africa, a degree of suppression of the immune system is commonplace. This creates a quite different immunological, epidemiological and clinical picture in Africa. For example, Kaposi's sarcoma, a tumour that was, before the arrival of Aids, only seen in the West among elderly Jews in Eastern and Central Europe, has long been common among much younger people in Central Africa.

In countries where funding for basic medical care is woefully inadequate, resources are simply not available for the painstaking epidemiological research into Aids that is required. What has happened is that a number of small and unreliable surveys in Africa have provided the basis for a mountain of dubious generalisation in the West.

A number of different factors may be involved in creating a more even distribution of Aids between the sexes in Africa, if indeed this proves to be the case. There may be a higher level of homosexual and bisexual activity than has been recognised. Heterosexual anal intercourse may play a part. The widespread re-use of non-sterile needles for immunisations, injections of antibiotics and other medications may also spread the infection. Whatever the case, it is impossible to generalise from Africa about the ways in which Aids may spread in the West.

Dr Brian Evans believes that Aids will remain a homosexual problem in Britain: 'Outside of Africa we have a handful of cases that might be by heterosexual transmission, yet here we are saying it's a heterosexual disease' (*Pulse,* 17 January 1987). The San Francisco Men's Health Study found that nearly half the homosexual and bisexual men tested were positive for the Aids virus, whereas all the heterosexual men were negative. Aids is undoubtedly a major health problem in parts of Central Africa, where it is spreading among men, women and children, and resources for treatment and research are urgently required. However, *there is no good evidence that Aids is likely to spread rapidly in the West among heterosexuals.*

Who can catch it?

'Any man or woman' can get the Aids virus, the government says; but this is true only if you engage in very specific forms of behaviour in very exclusive company. Men are at risk of picking up the Aids virus if they are the receptive partner in anal intercourse with an infected man. Women may be at risk if they have vaginal (or anal) intercourse with an infected man. And men or women drug users are at risk if they share needles or syringes with infected addicts. Haemophiliacs and recipients of blood transfusions need no longer be at risk: stocks of blood have been specially heat-treated to eliminate the virus.

The low infectiousness and remarkable fragility of the Aids virus—it can be killed by washing up liquid, moderate heat or dryness—mean that it is virtually exclusive to four limited social groups:

1. gay men living in a community in which the Aids virus has become established: that is, in any of the West's big-city scenes;
2. intravenous drug users in a similar community;
3. haemophiliacs or others who became infected through contaminated blood products before screening checks and heat treatment were introduced;
4. babies of mothers carrying the Aids virus: as neither gay men nor haemophiliacs (a disease which only affects men) bear children, in practice this means the babies of infected drug users.

From the arrival of the Aids virus in Britain in 1982 to the end of 1986, a total of 610 people developed Aids. Aids is concentrated in and around London—77 per cent of all cases have been reported to one of the four health authorities covering the capital and surrounding areas. Only handfuls of cases have been reported to other regional health authorities. The vast majority of people in Britain who do not fit into the four high-risk groups, or who do not live in the South-east, have little chance of catching the Aids virus—no matter what their sexual conduct.

'Aids is not just a homosexual disease' says the government's leaflet. But 88 per cent of the people who were diagnosed as having Aids in Britain up to the end of 1986 were male homosexuals. Adding the other risk categories brings the proportion to 97 per cent. In the USA, where the problem is much bigger, it is the same story—96 per cent of its 30 000 Aids cases fell into the four high-risk groups. The fact that, as the epidemic has spread in the USA, it has shown no tendency to extend beyond the main risk categories is powerful evidence of the low infectiousness of the virus.

Aids may not be 'prejudiced' against homosexuals, but right-wing politicians and moralists have seized on the association between Aids and homosexuality to whip up prejudice against gays. No matter how balanced the Aids leaflet pretends to be, it can only contribute to the anti-homosexual hysteria. However, it is striking that the government's leaflet downplays the anti-homosexual angle, in favour of playing up the minimal risks of the infection spreading among heterosexuals. More striking still is the way that many radicals, especially in the gay movement, have gone along with this approach. In their desire not to see gays singled out for blame, these radicals skate over the facts, encourage heterosexual anxieties and turn a blind eye to the mounting attack on homosexuals.

In noting that Aids predominantly affects gay men, we attribute no blame to them. On the contrary, this is our scientific point of departure for the defence of the rights of all homosexuals. When we acknowledge that anal intercourse is probably the major route by which the Aids virus has spread in the West, we recognise at the same time that millions of people the world over find this a pleasurable form of sexual activity. For us, clarifying the facts about Aids is the essential first step to tackling the real issues raised by the whole Aids scare—the denial of equal rights to homosexuals in our society and the attempt to take advantage of Aids to promote a general climate of sexual restraint.

Aids in perspective

Aids is indeed an incurable and fatal illness. By February 1987, the total of deaths from Aids in Britain had passed 350. This is a tragic loss of life, particularly because most of the deaths were of young people. But compared with other causes of death and disease, 350 deaths in four years is a marginal public health problem. In 1985 heart disease killed 190 000 people in Britain, cancer 134 000, and respiratory diseases 86 500. Car accidents kill around 5000 people, many of them children and young people, every year. Every year roughly 600 people die as a result of accidents at work—almost twice the number killed in four years by Aids. Another 800 people die each year as a result of occupational diseases such as pneumoconiosis (resulting from dust in coal mines and quarries), asbestosis (from asbestos used in lagging and construction) and byssinosis ('cotton dust disease').

There have been many alarmist projections about the spread of Aids in the future. Health minister Norman Fowler, for instance, is fond of quoting a figure of 4000 anticipated deaths over the next three years. The graph below shows the growth in Aids cases predicted by a widely used computer model—and the limits within which its predictions can be quoted with 95 per cent confidence of them being fulfilled (from *The Lancet,* 7 September 1985). According to this method the incidence of new cases of Aids in 1988 could be anywhere between 460 and 7300.

One critic has shown that, following this model through, every man, woman and child in Britain could have Aids by the year 2001 (see Nicholas Webb, *The Aids Virus: Forecasting Its Impact,* Office of Health Economics, December 1986). The advice of the model's authors, that its predictions 'should be interpreted with extreme caution', has been widely ignored. When given a range of possible figures of future Aids cases, politicians and the media always choose the highest and most alarming.

In the USA the exponential curve for the diffusion of Aids in 1982 and 1983 has already begun to flatten out. Such a pattern is typical of many biological phenomena. In the early stages the number of new cases of Aids in America doubled every five months, but this interval lengthened to 10 months in 1984-5 and to 11 months in 1985-6.

Fears about the rapid spread of Aids have been intensified by the widespread practice of publicising *cumulative totals* of those with the syndrome, rather than simply noting *new cases.* This creates steeply rising curves and general alarm. Studies of the spread of infectious diseases other than Aids generally rely on figures for new cases. These provide a more accurate assessment of the way that epidemics arise, grow and then die down. The difference is clear from the graphs below. In America, declining rates of diffusion of Aids are immediately apparent from the figures of new cases, but are obscured in the graph of cumulative totals. The same graph for Britain shows that the growth of new cases, while it has not yet levelled off, is much less alarming than the increase in the total number of Aids cases.

Just as the likely incidence of Aids *cases* has been exaggerated, there

The Aids epidemic in the USA

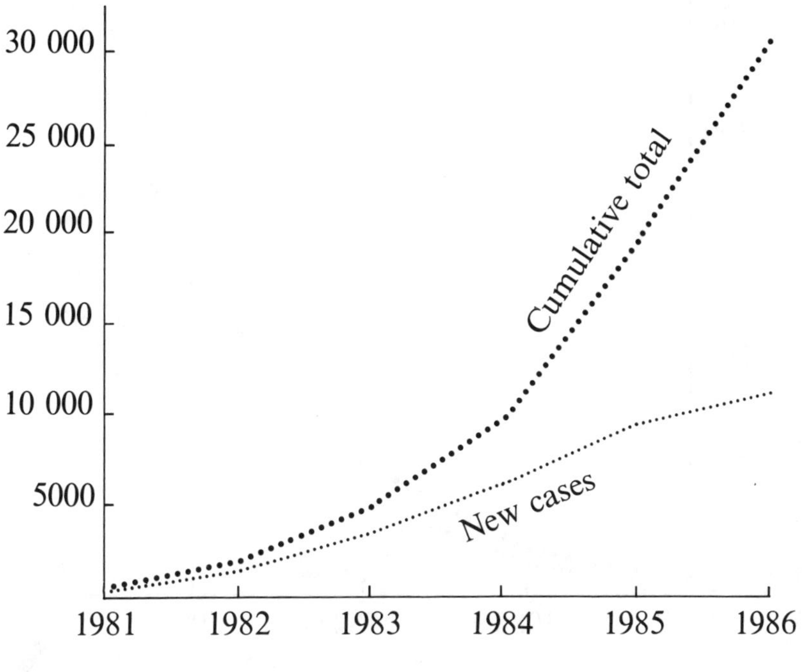

**Morbidity and
Mortality Weekly Reports, USA**

The Aids epidemic in Britain

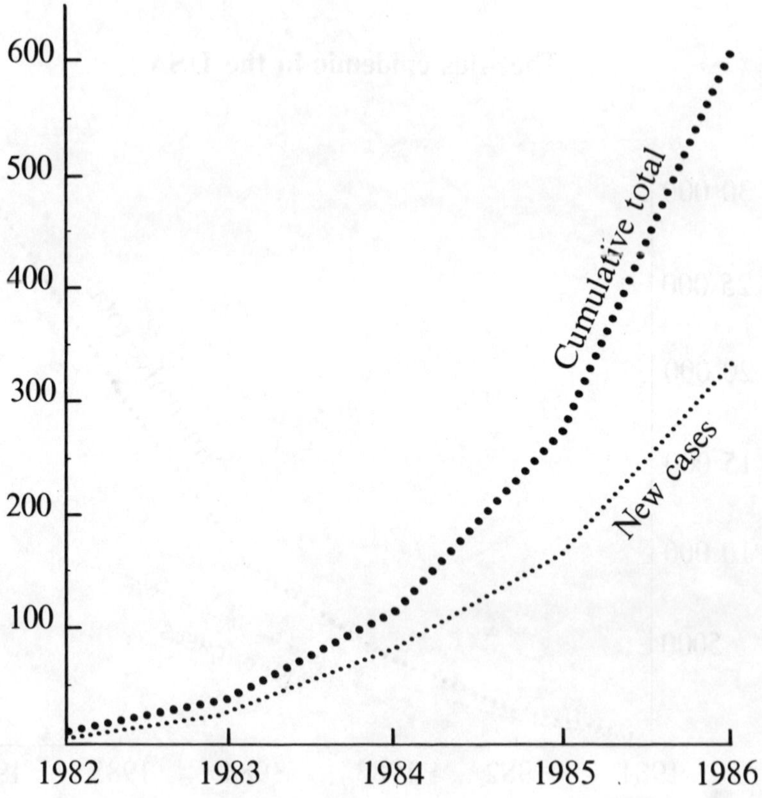

Compiled by
Communicable Diseases Surveillance Centre

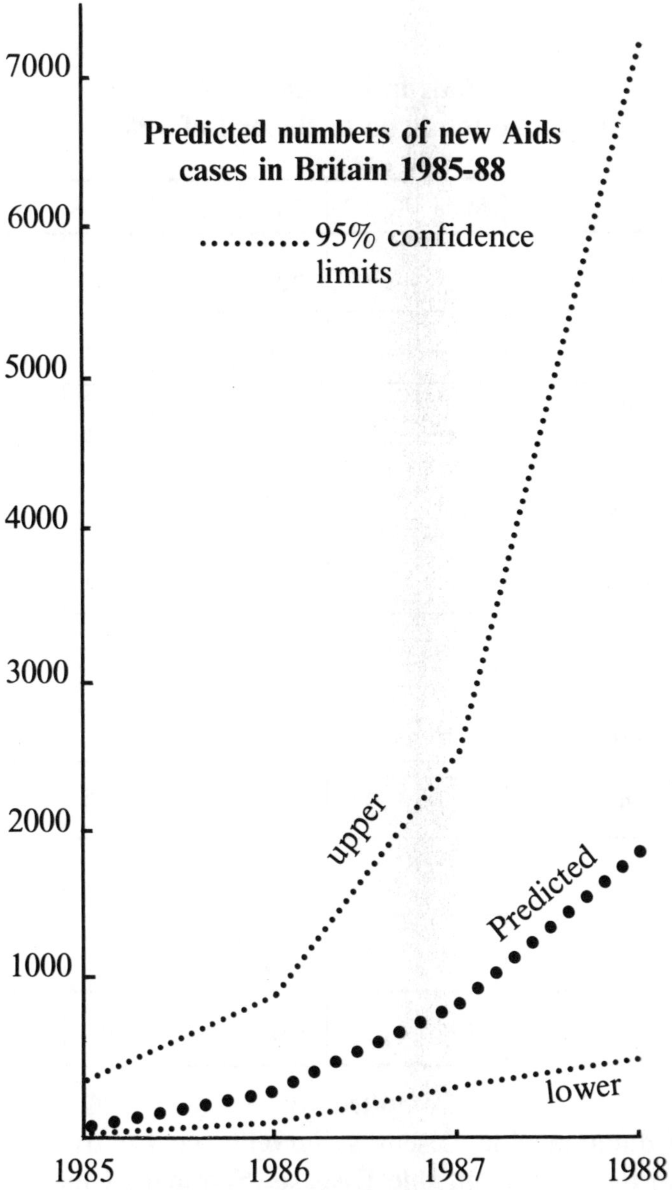

From *The Lancet,* 7 September 1985

Aids in Britain
Cumulative totals up to the end of 1986

	Male	Female	Total	%	Deaths	%
Homosexual/Bisexual	538	—	538	88	244	83
Intravenous drug abuser	7	2	9	1.5	2	0.7
Homosexual and IV drug abuser	6	0	6	1	4	1.4
Haemophiliac	25	—	25	4	19	7
Recipient of blood	6	4	10	2	9	3
Heterosexual:						
infected abroad	9	5	14	2	9	3
infected in Britain	1	3	4	0.7	3	1
Child of HIV+ mother	1	2	3	0.5	2	0.7
Other	—	1	1	0.2	1	0.3
Total	593	17	610	—	293	—

Compiled by
Communicable Diseases Surveillance Centre and the Communicable Disease (Scotland) Unit

are disturbing forecasts of the growth in the number of Aids *carriers.* These forecasts are often based on extrapolations from small surveys performed on unrepresentative populations such as drug addicts or those attending VD clinics. The government's widely quoted figure of 30 000 is little more than a guess. The only hard fact available in a welter of speculation is that 3105 positive antibody tests had been reported by July 1986. The screening of nearly two million blood donors between October 1985 and June 1986 revealed 41 to be HIV positive—a rate of 0.002 per cent ('Communicable Disease Report: Aids', July 1986). Subsequent interviews revealed that 90 per cent of these positives belonged to one of the four high-risk categories outlined above.

The number of people infected with the Aids virus is increasing, but the government's leaflet will not stop this rise by exhorting us all to 'take precautions'. Some precautions are obviously sensible for those in the high-risk categories—gay men in particular had been generally taking such measures on a growing scale long before the government launched its campaign (see *Capital Gay,* 3 October 1986, and *The Lancet,* 1 November 1986). For everybody else, special precautions are quite unnecessary.

'Why are you being sent this leaflet?'

Given the irrelevance of Aids to most people in Britain, this, the first question on the government's leaflet, is a fair one to ask. Here is the government's answer:

> 'This leaflet is being sent to every household in the country. It is about Aids. And everyone now needs to know the facts. It explains what the disease is. How it is spread. How serious a threat it is. And how it can be avoided.'

The government's offensive against Aids is the biggest and most costly health education campaign in British history. A special cabinet committee was set up to supervise it, with a budget of £20m for leaflets, posters, cinema and television commercials and a host of other publicity stunts. On the same November day that the Aids campaign was launched, the government quietly announced the abolition of the health education council. The council had annoyed the government by criticising cigarette companies and breweries that are an important source of state revenue and Conservative Party funds. So much for the Tories' commitment to health education!

The government has consistently refused to make more than

token gestures against today's preventable mass epidemics—coronary artery disease, lung cancer and alcoholism. Early detection can improve survival prospects in many forms of cancer. This is true of cancer of the cervix, which kills 2000 women every year and is a growing cause of death among younger women, and of breast cancer, which kills about 10 000 women every year. Yet the government has refused to provide the resources for properly organised screening facilities.

Everywhere the hypocrisy of the government over 'how serious a threat Aids is' is plain to see. The annual holocaust on the roads could be dramatically reduced by enforced speed limits of 50mph and a serious campaign against the drunken drivers who are responsible for many of the deaths. But such measures would antagonise the car manufacturers and the oil companies, as well as the big breweries and others engaged in the sale of alcohol. It would also cost money to make late night public transport a safe and reliable way for people to get home after having a few drinks.

Equally, the carnage on building sites, in coal mines, in factories and on North Sea oil rigs could be drastically reduced by ensuring that safety regulations were followed in every workplace. But in Britain today, the safety of workers takes second place to the drive to raise output and profits. That is why, at a time of rising industrial accidents, staff numbers at the government's embattled health and safety inspectorate are being cut back still further.

If the government were really concerned about the state of public health there are any number of campaigns it could launch. Yet of all the grave dangers facing the public, the government has chosen a rare disease—one which is spreading fairly slowly within certain clearly defined high-risk groups and which is unlikely, on current evidence, to spread very much further—to launch a propaganda blitz on every household in the nation.

A recent editorial in the *British Medical Journal* commented:

> 'HIV (the Aids virus) may well become endemic outside the current risk groups, but this could take years and may never be extensive. The question thus arises whether large sums of money earmarked for an advertising campaign might be better spent on improving treatment facilities or on basic research. An education campaign aimed at preventing the spread of HIV is, of course, to be welcomed provided that unnecessary fear is not provoked and that this rare disease is kept in perspective. Certainly, one could argue for more emphasis on the very low infectivity of the virus under normal circumstances and on the many ways by which it cannot be spread.' (3 January 1987)

 This rational assessment of the problem of Aids stands in marked contrast to the atmosphere of fear and prejudice that the government and the media have whipped up around the issue. In fact the government's emphasis is exactly the opposite of that called for here. The television commercial is full of images of death, and of doom-laden chimes and chants ('eerie electronic SFX', according to the script issued to the press). It is designed to frighten people into a return to conventional morality, and to deter all departures from this, such as homosexuality and promiscuity.

Before, however, we examine the *moral* aspect of the Aids panic, the more scientifically-minded reader may care to look more closely at the Aids virus and how it works. If you would prefer to skip the virology and the immunology, move straight to Chapter 3.

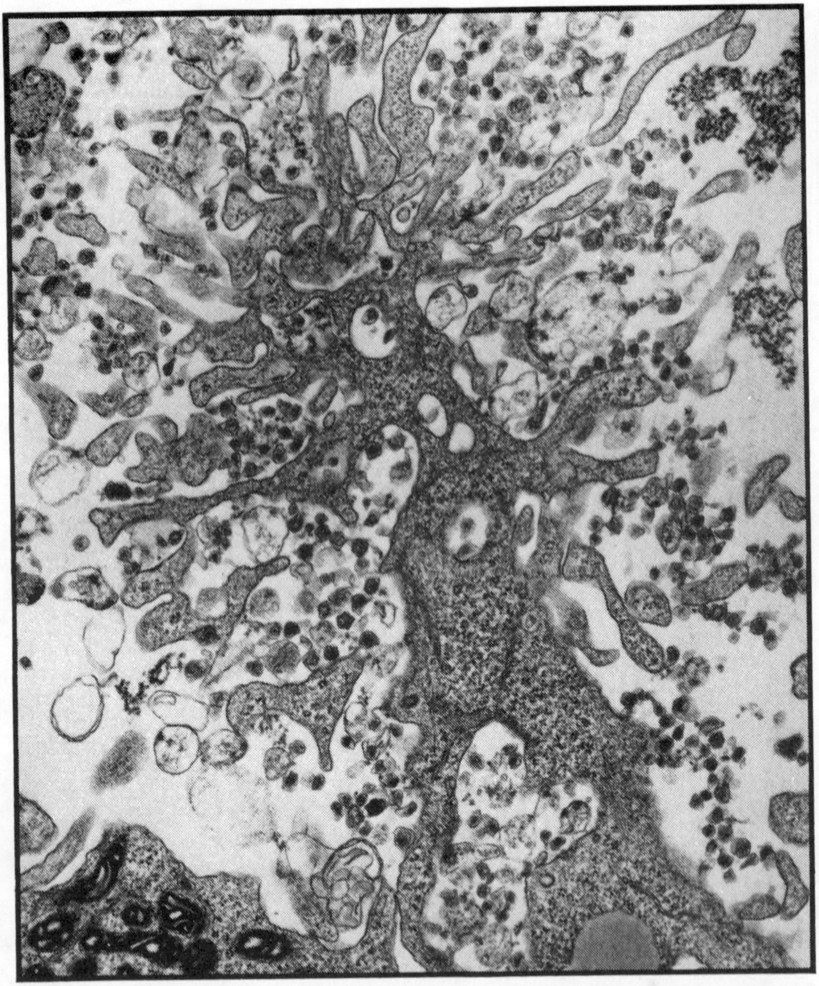

The onset of Aids: a T-cell explodes releasing a mass of newly-made particles of the Aids virus. The cell looks like a tree dying of Dutch elm disease: the virus particles are the small black specks.

2. How Aids works

The human immunodeficiency virus (HIV) that causes the acquired immune deficiency syndrome (Aids) is a remarkable beast. Unlike other parasites, from the organism which causes malaria through the plague bacillus to the virus which causes Lassa fever, the Aids virus does not kill its host directly. Rather, the Aids virus attacks the immune system, the human body's means of resisting all forms of infection. It kills by rendering its victim vulnerable to parasites which any healthy person would easily fight off.

The immune system

To understand Aids it is necessary to grasp the basics of the immune system. The human body has two mechanisms for resisting infection: one is inborn, the other is acquired through exposure to potentially harmful organisms.

Inborn mechanisms for deterring and destroying invaders provide the front line of resistance to infection. Skin—thick, dry and tough—keeps out all but the most well-adapted parasites. By contrast, the thin, warm and moist linings covering the digestive, respiratory and reproductive tracts provide less protection and are the most common portals of entry for disease organisms. These surfaces are, however, defended both by specialised cells and by anti-septic secretions—such as tears, saliva and stomach acid.

The body's second line of defence is the immunity acquired through experience of infection. The evolution of human society is in many ways the history of the development of acquired immunity to parasites (see William H McNeill, *Plagues and Peoples,* 1977). Modern immunology has shown that lymphocytes—specialised white blood cells produced in the bone marrow and circulating in the blood and lymphatic systems—play the central role in enabling the body to recognise and combat foreign invaders.

The system of acquired immunity has two components: cellular and humoral. The key agents in *cellular* immunity are specialised lymphocytes called T-cells. T-cells are controlled by the thymus gland, which is located in the chest, above the heart. They recognise and respond to the presence of foreign micro-organisms. Each T-cell reacts specifically to a particular component, known as the antigen, on the surface of an alien bacterium or virus.

Different types of T-cells respond differently. 'Helper' T-cells activate other specialised lymphocytes—B-cells—to produce antibodies, complex proteins called immunoglobulins, which help to neutralise the antigen by sticking to it. 'Suppressor' T-cells regulate the production of antibody and turn it off when the threat has subsided. 'Killer' T-cells directly attack and destroy invaders. Other specialised white blood cells—macrophages and monocytes—play a similar role to killer T-cells.

Humoral immunity results from the presence of antibodies circulating in the blood stream and in other body fluids, or 'humours'. When activated by helper T-cells, B-cells pump out immunoglobulins which stick on to the enemy antigens and render them susceptible to attack by killer T-cells and macrophages.

Because the immune system is so vital to human life, malfunctions tend to have grave consequences. Inborn deficiencies in the system are rare and rapidly fatal. The most familiar form of acquired immune deficiency results from the use of cytotoxic (literally 'cell-poisoning') drugs to prevent the body from rejecting alien tissue in the form of heart, kidney or other organ transplants. A similar state of immune suppression results from the use of cytotoxic drugs and radiotherapy in the treatment of certain cancers. Any extreme stress—such as trauma, burns, or major illness—may have a similar effect. Certain chronic infections and the use of intravenous drugs seem also to suppress the immune response.

However, by far the most common *acquired* cause of a malfunctioning immune system is malnutrition, a condition which is estimated to afflict half a billion people worldwide. Starvation causes the thymus gland to waste, leading to defects in all T-cell functions. This is undoubtedly an important factor in the spread of Aids in Central Africa, where famine is widespread.

The virus

The Aids virus is a tiny strand of RNA, the basic chain of chemicals through which all forms of organic life replicate themselves, surrounded by a membrane of fatty material. It is, as we have noted, very fragile. However, if HIV succeeds in getting into the human body, it has an affinity for a particular antigen-receptor site (T4) on helper T-cells. Mistaking HIV for something familiar, the T-cell sticks to it and the virus gains entry into the cell. It then rapidly loses its coat and releases its single strand of RNA inside the cell.

The agent which causes Aids is a human retrovirus, a group only discovered over the past decade. What makes the retrovirus distinctive is that, once it has entered the cell, it multiplies by transcribing itself into double-stranded DNA which is incorporated into the DNA of the host cell. It thus takes over the cell, which can now produce copies of the virus. This is the opposite of the usual process in which DNA acts as a template for the production of RNA. The retroviruses can do this because they possess the unique biological catalyst *reverse transcriptase.*

Once the DNA produced by the virus—pro-viral DNA—has been incorporated into the host cell's DNA, it may remain latent for a period of time. During this period an infected person is an Aids carrier, with HIV in blood, semen and other body fluids. But the person remains well, without any of the symptoms of fully developed Aids. This latent period comes to an abrupt end when the lymphocytes which are playing host to the Aids virus are stimulated—possibly in response to some additional infection. 'Then', as one expert account describes the critical stage in the development of Aids, 'the virus bursts into action, reproducing itself so furiously that the new virus particles escaping from the cell riddle the cellular membrane with holes and the lymphocyte dies' (see Robert C Gallo, 'The Aids Virus', *Scientific American,* January 1987).

The Aids virus seems to hit T-helper cells the hardest: a declining ratio of T-helper to T-suppressor cells is a characteristic feature of the infection. However, the virus also attacks other T-cells, B-cells and macrophages, steadily paralysing the whole immune system. The virus also appears to attach itself directly to brain cells, producing neurological damage which may culminate in dementia in a minority of Aids patients.

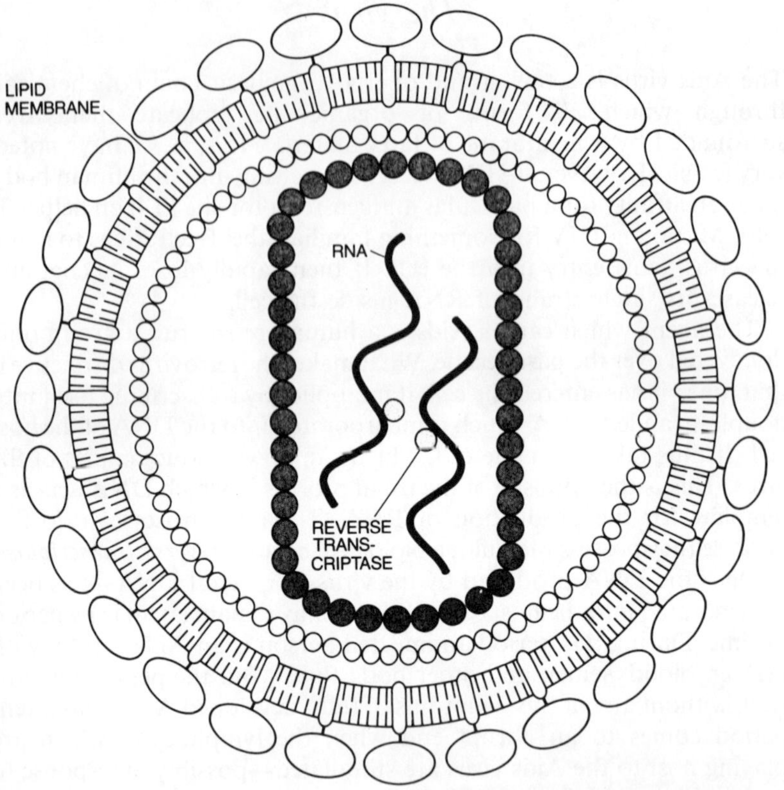

The Aids virus: a particle one ten-thousandth of a millimetre across. The virus is covered by a membrane made up of two layers of lipid (fatty) material studded with glycoproteins (proteins with attached sugar chains). The viral RNA is surrounded by a core made up of proteins: each strand of RNA carries several copies of the enzyme reverse transcriptase which catalyses the assembly of the viral DNA. (from **Scientific American,** ***January 1987)***

The retroviruses were first discovered in animals, in which they appear to be responsible for a range of tumours and disorders of the immune system. The cat leukaemia virus, sometimes called the feline Aids virus, is now considered to be one of the commonest causes of death in the domestic cat. The first human retrovirus to be discovered, which was named Human T-cell Leukaemia Virus Type 1, was found to be the causative agent of a rare type of leukaemia confined to certain parts of the USA, Central Africa and Japan. The second–HTLV Type 2—was isolated from two patients suffering another rare form of leukaemia, but it seemed not to be the causative agent.

The virus that causes Aids was first identified by Luc Montagnier, Francoise Barré-Sinoussi and Jean-Claude Chermann at the Pasteur Institute in Paris in 1983. They named it LAV—the Lymphadenopathy-Associated Virus—because the most prominent clinical feature in those infected was swelling of the lymph glands. In 1984 Robert Gallo and his co-workers at the National Institutes of Health at Bethesda identified in Aids patients an agent they called HTLV Type 3—Human T-cell Lymphotrophic Virus Type 3. This terminology reflected their observation that the virus selectively attacked T-cells. Despite an unseemly wrangle among the scientists over who named the virus first, it soon became apparent that the French and American teams were talking about the same beast. In 1986, by common international agreement, it was renamed HIV.

The Aids virus has two other significant features. It is highly unstable in its basic genetic structure, leading to considerable variations in the form of the virus isolated from different patients. In this respect it resembles the influenza virus, which regularly reappears in different strains; like flu, Aids is a disease for which the development of an effective vaccine is likely to prove particularly difficult.

The second feature of HIV is that it provokes the body to produce a specific antibody. While this appears to have no effect in helping to neutralise the virus, it is useful in demonstrating exposure to it; indeed this phenomenon provides the basis for the HIV antibody test. Antibodies usually appear within eight weeks of infection, though this process of 'seroconversion' may be delayed for several months. However, positive antibody status—being 'body positive'—provides no guide to the size of the viral challenge nor to the likely prognosis for the infected individual.

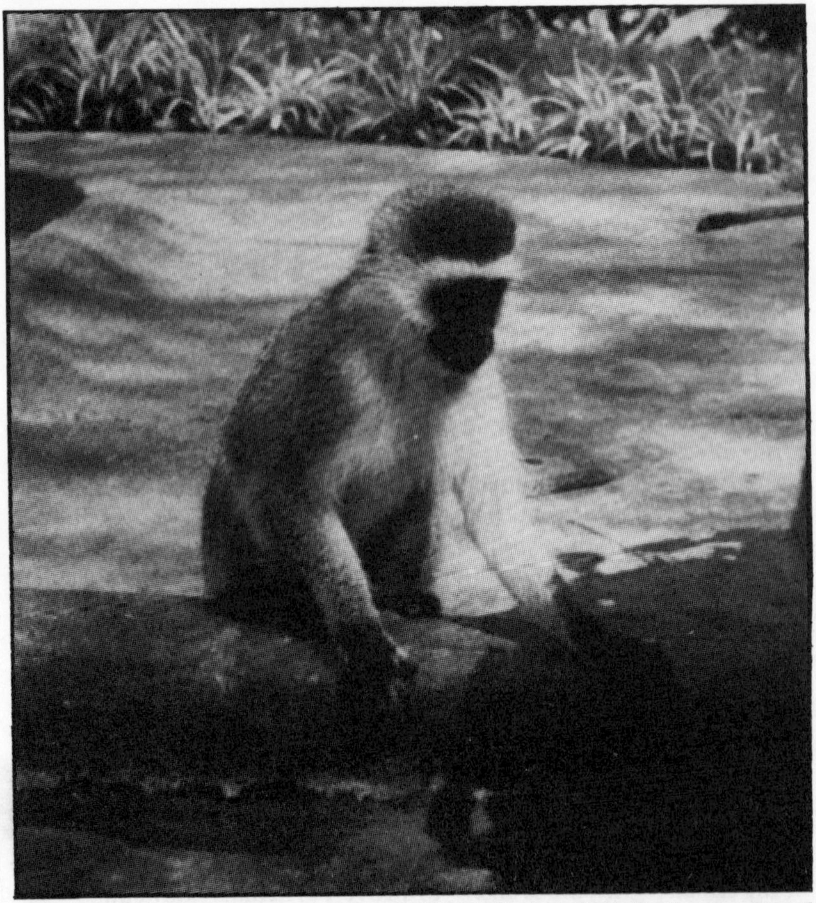

The African green monkey: the host of STLV-III, thought to be the ancestor of the Aids virus. (from Scientific American, ***January 1987)***

Aids was labelled a syndrome because, when it was first recognised in 1981, it was seen as a collection of symptoms and signs of disease for which no clear cause could be identified. The name has stuck even though the causative organism was soon discovered. Indeed the speed of advance of medical understanding of Aids has been remarkable. The Aids virus was identified within three years of the first description of the mysterious syndrome and a reliable screening test based on detecting antibodies to HIV was available shortly afterwards. The first treatment for Aids—azidothymidine or AZT—is already undergoing intensive trials, and research into a vaccine is well underway.

What effect does the Aids virus have on its victims? A number of inter-related disease states have been clearly associated with HIV infection.

- **Acute retroviral illness**

Between four and 12 weeks after exposure to HIV, there may be an acute illness characterised by symptoms similar to those associated with glandular fever. The patient feels tired and unwell, complains of a sore throat and aching muscles, and has a fever, swollen glands and a rash. These symptoms usually clear up within two weeks. During the course of this illness the HIV test becomes positive. In most cases, however, HIV infection produces no such acute illness.

- **Persistent generalised lymphadenopathy**

Roughly 30 per cent of those with HIV infection develop lymphadenopathy—swelling of the lymph glands around the neck, armpits and groin. This must be present for at least three months to justify the diagnosis. Most people with persistent generalised lymphadenopathy do not feel unwell, though some complain of constant fatigue. Some sufferers apparently revert to a healthy state as carriers of HIV.

- **Aids-related complex**

The development of Aids-related complex marks a significant deterioration in the patient's immune system. It is characterised by prolonged fever (more than two months), chronic diarrhoea (more than one month), severe weight loss (more than 10 per cent), and persistent malaise and lethargy. There may also be persistent generalised lymphadenopathy and an enlarged liver and spleen. An increased susceptibility to infection is revealed by the onset of oral thrush, shingles and boils.

- **Aids**

On the basis of current knowledge, it appears that between 10 and 15 per cent of those infected with HIV progress from any of the above conditions to full-blown Aids within three years. The diagnosis of Aids is indicated by the development of opportunist infections—notably pneumocystis carinii pneumonia—or of tumours, especially Kaposi's sarcoma of the skin. Such conditions are very rare except in patients whose immune system is suppressed. Aids sufferers are prone to infection with a wide range of protozoa, fungi, bacteria and viruses that are normally harmless to man. They are also vulnerable to uncommon tumours, particularly of the lymphatic tissue.

Aids is fatal. While in the early stages it is possible to treat infections with antibiotics, the progressive destruction of the immune system makes for a losing battle. The overall median survival time of Aids patients in Britain has been calculated to be 13.5 months (*British Medical Journal,* 28 June 1986). Within 28 months of detection, 75 per cent of British Aids sufferers were dead.

The epidemic

An epidemic is said to exist when the incidence of new cases of a disease exceeds normal expectations. The peculiarity of Aids has been the rising numbers of new cases of an entirely new disease. This has given a certain plausibility to theories which put the disease down to the release of an artificially manufactured virus from some centre of biological warfare. Such theories have been proposed by recognised scientific authorities such as Medvedev and Seale. British astronomer Fred Hoyle still sticks to his theory of an extra-terrestrial origin for the epidemic. However, more mundane explanations are quite adequate to account for the emergence of the Aids virus.

The most likely story is that HIV has recently jumped from an animal to a human host, perhaps adapting its structure with all the subtlety of which it is known to be capable. This route has supplied human societies with most of their familiar infectious diseases, such as measles, mumps, whooping cough, smallpox, tuberculosis, typhus and the plague.

There are several recent examples of infections which have suddenly crossed over from animals to man. In 1959 the virus causing O'nyong nyong fever passed from monkeys to man in Uganda, causing a short-lived epidemic. In 1967 laboratory workers in Marburg, West Germany, became infected with a viral illness contracted from Ugandan vervet monkeys on which they were conducting experiments. Lassa fever originated in rodents in Nigeria and was first diagnosed in man in 1969. In a susceptible human population, such new infections often spread rapidly, causing a high level of fatalities, before they are brought under control.

The origins of human immunoviruses

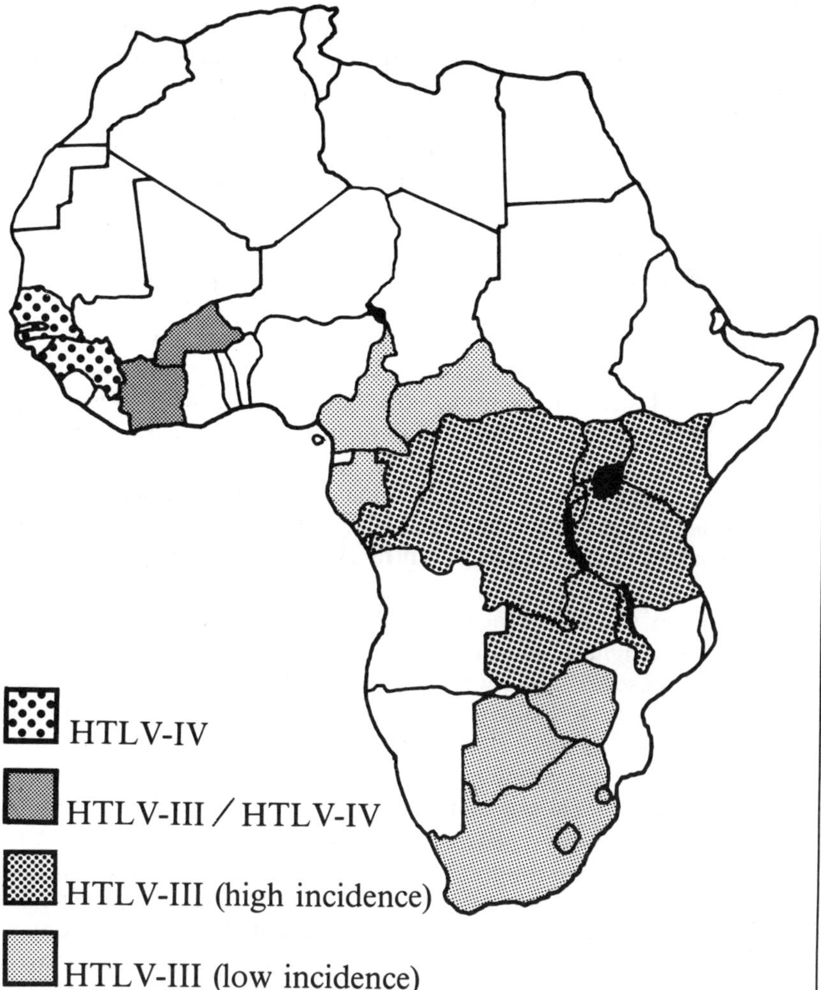

Studies in Africa in 1985 and early 1986 show the highest rates of HTLV-III (HIV) infection in a band across central Africa, with lower rates in areas to the north and south. The map also shows the distribution of HTLV-IV, a virus intermediate between HTLV III and the monkey Aids virus STLV-III, which appears not to cause disease in man. (from **Scientific American,** ***January 1987)***

The case for an animal origin for Aids has been strengthened by the discovery of viruses very similar to HIV in the Asian macacque monkey and in the African green monkey. A virus labelled Simian T-cell Lymphotrophic Virus causes an Aids-like illness among monkeys in North American zoos.

It is possible that the Aids virus passed from monkeys to man in some part of Africa and then remained confined for a time to some remote population. However, over the past decade the increased mobility of people in Africa, in conditions of widespread poverty, malnutrition and chronic infection with other diseases, may have helped to spread HIV. The general drift towards the city and the breakdown of traditional constraints on sexual behaviour may have accelerated the diffusion of the virus. The widespread use of contaminated needles for immunisation and medication may also have played a part.

The increased scale of international travel may have helped to extend HIV infection around the world, just as camel caravans, sailboats and steamships spread the infectious epidemics of earlier epochs. Sexual contact between American tourists and local people in Central Africa seems to have been the main route through which the virus made its way to the USA. It remains unclear whether Aids was transmitted to the Caribbean island state of Haiti by American tourists or by workers exchanged with Central African states in the sixties and seventies. Aids came to Europe both indirectly, from the USA, and directly from Central Africa, leading to high levels of infection in France and Belgium, countries with close links to the region.

The first cases of Aids were noted in the USA in 1981, when the Centers for Disease Control in Atlanta, Georgia, noted a dramatic increase in the incidence of pneumocystis carinii pneumonia and Kaposi's sarcoma in young men. By the end of 1981 some 252 cases of Aids had been diagnosed in the USA; by the end of 1985, close to 19 000 cases had been registered, and 9000 people were already dead. Aids had become a common cause of death among young men in a number of big cities: San Francisco, New York and Miami were the most prominent. In London, the Communicable Disease Surveillance Centre noted a similar trend. Britain's first three cases were diagnosed in 1982; by February 1987 the number was 686 of whom 355 were already dead.

As a new, fatal and sexually transmitted disease that mainly affected gay men, Aids seemed tailor-made for Western moralists. Whether or not they manufactured it in some secret laboratory, they soon turned Aids into a powerful propaganda weapon.

3. Moral panics

'Societies appear to be subject, every now and then, to periods of moral panic,' wrote the sociologist Stanley Cohen in 1972. Cohen outlined the character of a moral panic as follows:

> 'A condition, episode, person or group of persons emerges to become defined as a threat to societal values and interests; its nature is presented in a stylised and stereotypical fashion by the mass media; the moral barricades are manned by editors, bishops, politicians and other right-thinking people; socially accredited experts pronounce their diagnoses and solutions; ways of coping are evolved or (more often) resorted to.' (*Folk Devils and Moral Panics,* 1972)

Cohen's book focused on the moral panic generated around the excursions of 'mods and rockers' to seaside towns on bank holiday weekends, and on other manifestations of the new 'youth culture' of the mid-sixties. His study also refers to 'parallel reactions to the drug problem, student militancy, political demonstrations, football hooliganism, vandalism of various kinds and crime and violence in general'. It is notable that panics over virtually all these issues rage with renewed intensity today. Only student militancy is now missing from a list which Cohen drew up all of 15 years ago. We can add mugging, child abuse, picket line violence, international terrorism—and Aids—as new subjects for national hysteria.

Cohen's strength is his refusal to take at face value the images of social deviancy as presented by the mass media. His weakness is that he fails to take into account the wider historical context within which a moral panic takes place. Thus he can with impunity draw parallels between 'crime waves' in seventeenth-century Massachusetts, the furore over marijuana-smoking among American youths in the thirties, and the post-war panic over 'teddy boys' in South London.

The moral panics of the sixties took place in a society in which economic expansion and political consensus encouraged a climate of liberalism. This meant that panics could come and go without causing much more disruption than a bank holiday traffic jam. In crisis-stricken modern Britain, by contrast, a similar sort of moral panic—for example, the fuss about the Stonehenge hippies in summer 1986—leads to the despatch of fully equipped riot squads, mass arrests, beatings and imprisonments, and to the wholesale confiscation of vehicles.

In a period of social crisis a moral panic can have much broader consequences than is evident from Cohen's superficial parallels between diverse small-scale social upheavals. One example of a moral panic which had a lasting impact on world politics was the West's crusade against communism in the late forties and early fifties.

In those years, the threats to Western values were defined as the Soviet Union abroad and communists, communist sympathisers, left wingers, trade union activists and even liberals at home. A generation of red-baiting politicians, personified by Senator Joseph McCarthy in the USA, tracked down the communist menace in every walk of life—in the civil service, the unions, in the media and in education. Press, trade union, labour and church leaders all played an active part in promoting the panic and carrying out purges. While the Cold War witch-hunt was most ferocious in the USA, left wingers were victimised and intimidated in every Western country.

A series of sensational cases featuring Soviet spies, traitors and defectors dominated the headlines: the trial and execution of the Rosenbergs in the USA, the defections of Burgess and Maclean from Britain, the Gouzenko scandal in Canada and the Petrov affair in Australia. Communists were elevated into a major threat to every decent God-fearing citizen and patriot. Repressive laws, official inquisitions and the widespread use of undercover police agents were all justified by the need to protect society against 'the reds'. Public confessions and denunciations, oaths of loyalty and the censorship of books and films were also deployed.

The mentality created by the Cold War had a number of features which, as we shall see, are shared by the Aids panic.

• Rationality and irrationality

A major moral panic needs a basic element of logic around which irrational fears can be stirred up. At the close of the Second World War, the strength of mass anti-capitalist sentiments and sympathy for the Soviet Union was a real problem for the authorities. At a time when the Soviet Union was consolidating its hold on Eastern Europe, it was vital for Western rulers to tighten their grip at home. Anti-communism provided the means of achieving this objective.

In fact, the West was never in jeopardy in the late forties. Only the Greek, Italian and French communist parties had mass influence, and they rapidly subordinated themselves to the new post-war order. Significantly, it was where the left was weakest—in the USA, Canada, Australia and Britain—that irrational fears of the communist menace gained the greatest influence. The feebleness of working class politics in the English-speaking world allowed anti-working class prejudices to spread with a feverish intensity.

• Consensus and diversion

One of the most important consequences of a successful moral panic is that it both rallies a wide consensus of support behind the establishment on the issue at stake, and also diverts attention from more immediate social and political problems. The Cold War forged a great spirit of common purpose in the West, both internationally (formation of the Nato alliance, etc) and nationally (era of witch-hunts in the unions, blacklisting and so on).

Unity and 'security' against Stalin and against communist subversion at home were fundamental to the post-war social order. Fingering 'the communists' meant that the austerity conditions of wartime could be prolonged to allow the revival of the Western capitalist economies.

• Repression and reaction

Major moral panics help create a climate favourable to repressive measures—measures which affect not only the target group concerned, but also much wider sections of society. The crusade against communism in the USA led to the victimisation of tens of thousands of workers in the federal civil service and in state and municipal government. Thousands more were driven out of jobs in the newspapers, in Hollywood, and in schools and universities. Even in Britain hundreds were purged from the civil service by Attlee's Labour government.

Organised labour was the main target of wider repression. In the USA the Cold War put an abrupt end to the trade union militancy of the mid-forties. The Taft-Hartley Act allowed state interference in labour relations and union affairs; Congress 'investigated' the unions; and the Loyalty-Security Program, first introduced in the civil service, was soon extended to cover all industries holding defence contracts.

The most lasting defeat of the Cold War lay, however, in the way the American labour movement succumbed to anti-communist prejudice:

> 'The Cold War penetrated directly into working class life and its organisations, and it did so by a combination of selective coercion and material incentives. Ideologically, the effect was devastating for progressive politics in America.' (Reg Whitaker, 'Fighting the Cold War on the Home Front: America, Britain, Australia and Canada', in *The Socialist Register*, 1984)

The intensified oppression of homosexuals in all Western countries was one significant outcome of Cold War ideology.

Why the Aids scare now?

Sex, disease, death: Aids is an ideal focus for a moral panic today. The scope for stirring up public anxieties, fears and animosities is enormous. The Aids epidemic hit the USA in 1981, shortly after a newly elected Ronald Reagan opened a new era of austerity, militarism and narrow-mindedness. It arrived in Britain in 1982, the year of the Falklands War, a year of armed aggression abroad and rampant chauvinism at home. Yet it was not until 1986 that the British establishment really launched the Aids panic. After all the promises of recovery, another year of economic decay exposed the failure of the Thatcher government to halt the collapse of the British economy and pushed it into a more openly political offensive against its opponents.

As a general election looms, the Tories have compensated for their vulnerability on economic matters by dwelling on issues such as terrorism, national security, law and order, drugs, child abuse and crime—issues which they know put the opposition parties on the defensive. At a time of deepening social crisis, the government has now thrown its full weight behind the Aids panic, the most subtle and in many ways the most successful moral panic ever sponsored in Britain.

To many, the government campaign for what it calls 'safe sex' appears a rational response to the serious problems thrown up by the Aids virus. Let's look at the safe sex campaign more closely.

4. The dangers of safe sex

'Do you think this caring government would swap my Aids leaflet (as new) for a bucket of coal?' asked an elderly woman living alone in Dorset in a letter to a national newspaper in January. Posting the official Aids leaflet to every household in Britain in the coldest January for decades summed up the absurdity of the safe sex campaign. About a third of the homes receiving the leaflet contained either a single person over 60, or an elderly couple. For the millions of pensioners who learnt the importance of shunning promiscuity and using condoms, hypothermia was a much more serious threat to life.

Government publicity is, in the view of more zealous campaigners against Aids, not explicit or chilling enough in its warnings against various sexual practices. In fact, however, the scale of the government's propaganda is out of all proportion to the real dangers.

As we have seen, Aids is rare in Britain. Furthermore, infection is virtually exclusive to certain high-risk categories. The danger of the virus spreading beyond these groups, by heterosexual intercourse, has been grossly exaggerated. The anti-Aids commercial shown to Scottish television viewers, which depicted members of a single family disappearing one by one, was grotesquely alarmist. Special instructions issued by the authorities to Scottish schools about the dangers of children pricking their fingers and using their own blood in classroom experiments are quite absurd. In communities where the prevalence of the Aids virus is almost certainly zero, children can engage in the most extravagant blood-mixing rituals without the slightest risk of catching Aids.

Aids is a real health risk in Britain to homosexual men who have repeatedly engaged in unprotected receptive anal intercourse, particularly in the London area, over the past couple of years. It is a risk, too, to intravenous drug users who have shared their needles with other users in London or Edinburgh over the same period. Apart from these fairly clearly defined groups, HIV infection is not at present a serious health problem.

A bogus solution

While the safe sex campaign may cause widespread alarm among people who have a higher chance of being run over by a bus than they have of contracting Aids, it will not stop the spread of Aids in the high-risk categories.

'The more sexual partners you have, especially male partners, the more chance you have of having sex with someone who is infected' explains the government leaflet. Within the London gay scene, where there are undoubtedly many HIV-positive men, this may well be true. Yet, given a rising level of HIV infection in this social group, reducing the number of your sexual partners will not necessarily reduce the risk to you. For example, if a gay man reduces the number of his partners in the course of a year from 10 to three, while the prevalence of HIV infection rises from 10 to 33 per cent, the man's chances of having sex with an infected partner remain the same.

The defect of the safe sex campaign as a means of preventing the spread of HIV infection among gay men is that it fails to take into account the dominant feature in the life of homosexuals—the fact that they are oppressed.

The inequality of homosexuals is set out in Acts of parliament and enforced by the courts. The 1967 Sexual Offences Act is widely regarded as having legalised homosexuality in Britain. In fact it legalised what nobody was ever caught for—sexual relations in private between 'consenting adults' (men over the age of 21). In fact it made it easier for the police to secure convictions for other forms of homosexual activity.

Lord Arran, who drew up the Act, summed up the prevailing attitude: 'I ask those who have, as it were, been in bondage and for whom the prison doors are now open to show their thanks by comporting themselves quietly and with dignity' (quoted in Jeffrey

Weeks, *Coming Out: Homosexual Politics in Britain from the Nineteenth Century to the Present,* 1977). In the years immediately following the Act the number of prosecutions actually increased. Had Oscar Wilde come to trial in 1968, instead of 1895, he would have been liable for a maximum sentence of five years instead of two.

In addition to the 1967 Act, homosexuals are discriminated against by a wide range of other criminal and civil legislation. Gay men are commonly prosecuted for gross indecency, for importuning and, under public order laws, for simply holding hands or kissing in public places. The use of plainclothes police as agents provocateurs is commonplace under certain police authorities. In divorce settlements and in disputes over custody of children, lesbians and gay men receive unequal treatment at the prejudiced discretion of the courts. The criminalisation of homosexuality provides the legal backing for a much wider pattern of discrimination and harassment.

People who are known to be lesbian or gay confront rigorous discrimination at work. This takes the form of constant gibes and petty harassment from fellow workers, which make it easy for employers to get away with victimising homosexual workers. Most lesbians and gays deal with this by concealing their sexual orientation. Often, they are forced to go along with the prevailing climate of hatred towards homosexuals—even to the extent of establishing, or inventing, heterosexual relationships which can be produced in response to probing questions and office gossip.

A minority of lesbians and gays deal with the workplace by allowing their homosexuality to become a sort of open secret. Selected workmates and even employers become aware of it, but the homosexual person keeps a low profile. In big cities, this arrangement is commonplace in the professions—among teachers, social workers, and so on. It works well—as long as nothing happens that requires an explicit recognition of sexual orientation.

Some homosexuals are able to find work in jobs in which they are not obliged to conceal their sexuality—in the offices of radical Labour councils, for example. Others simply perform as gay barman, actor or nurse; women prison officers and male hairdressers, for instance, have in their work a kind of stereotyped leeway as homosexuals. Whatever survival strategy individual lesbians or gay men adopt, however, it is evident that their access to employment and their promotion prospects are sharply circumscribed by their sexuality.

Discrimination in employment is reinforced by discrimination in wider society. Homosexuals cannot go about together without constantly being alert to the reactions they might encounter. They cannot hold hands in public or chat too intimately in most pubs or public places. They cannot freely court, dance together, whisper sweet nothings at bus stops, or kiss goodbye at railway stations or airports. Homosexuals are forced to live like escaped convicts in straight society.

The penalties for breaking out, or for being found out as homosexual, are swift and often savage. Ridicule, disgrace, the sack, eviction or a beating are all commonplace experiences. These responses are made respectable by the law and are enforced by the police, magistrates, social workers, probation officers, doctors, teachers—and by an army of self-appointed queer-bashers.

There are therefore two broad categories of male homosexuals. There are those who have come out and are openly gay at home, at work and in their social and sexual life. There are also other gay men who, fearing rejection, discrimination and repression, have not openly declared their sexual identity to their families, workmates and friends. They are forced to conduct their homosexual relationships in a more or less secretive and insecure way. According to all researches into sexual behaviour in modern society, the overwhelming majority of gay men, especially those who are working class, young or black, belong to the second category.

For the gay minority who have come out, the government's safe sex campaign is *unnecessary.* Over the past couple of years VD clinics throughout the Western world have recorded a sharp decline in venereal diseases—most notably of rectal gonorrhoea, which is contracted through anal intercourse. The figures suggest that the use of condoms has already become widespread among sexually active gay men. This has little to do with safe sex advertising, and much more with gay men recognising the consequences of HIV infection once the impact of Aids on the American gay scene became widely known in 1983 and 1984.

For the majority of gay men who are forced to pursue their homosexual encounters furtively, campaigns for safe sex are *useless.* The clandestine and chancy circumstances in which most gay men conduct their sexual encounters make it difficult for them to follow the government's guidelines in practice. The climate of guilt, secrecy and fear that surrounds much homosexual activity in Britain creates the conditions in which the Aids virus can flourish.

It is the *oppression of homosexuals* that allows HIV infection to spread among gay men. Hence, the way to stop the spread of Aids is neither to pretend that it is a threat to heterosexuals, nor to make futile exhortations to gays, but rather to challenge *every* act of discrimination or harassment directed against homosexuals.

The other high-risk group in which the Aids virus may spread is intravenous drug users. Yet the authorities have consistently prevaricated over giving official support for the simplest preventive measure—the issue of free disposable needles and syringes. The authorities' bizarre argument against this proposal is that providing sterile equipment to inject drugs will encourage people to take up intravenous drug abuse. In fact this conflict between two of the establishment's favourite panics—drugs and Aids—simply shows that the government is more interested in using these social problems for their wider scare value than it is in taking practical measures to prevent the spread of HIV infection.

How VD was curbed

The drive to control venereal disease in the past provides an interesting parallel with the campaign against Aids today. The parallel is not exact because, unlike Aids, syphilis and gonorrhoea were as easily spread by heterosexuals as homosexuals; female prostitutes, for example, were a major pool of infection. In the late nineteenth and early twentieth centuries, the British government introduced a number of repressive laws aimed at curbing an epidemic of VD.

Under the Contagious Diseases Prevention Act of 1864, prostitutes could be forcibly detained for up to three months for medical treatment. Similar measures were introduced under the Defence of the Realm Act during the First World War, when a woman could be imprisoned for six months for infecting a member of the armed forces with VD. The authorities supplemented state terror with endless sermons on the virtues of chastity and purity.

Both repression and exhortation proved ineffective in reducing VD. It became a major public health problem, causing blindness in babies, high levels of infertility, dementia and death. The gradual decline in VD in the inter-war years can be attributed in part to the general improvement in the position of women in society which followed the struggle for the vote. The parallel improvement in women's economic position reduced the number of women driven on to the streets to make a living. There was also some relaxation in the harassment of prostitutes by the police and the courts.

The partial decriminalisation of prostitution following the repeal of the Contagious Diseases and the Defence of the Realm Acts contributed to the success of the special treatment clinics for VD set up after the First World War. The removal of some of the stigma attached to VD encouraged sufferers to attend and also made it possible for confidential contact-tracing to take place. The discovery of specific antibiotics for treating the main venereal diseases during the Second World War made it possible to reduce drastically the incidence of VD.

The modern response to Aids recalls the debate about how to curb VD. On the one hand there is the safe sex campaign. On the other, there are strident calls for the re-introduction of something like the Contagious Diseases Act. For example, Tony Lester, a Tory councillor in Edinburgh, has demanded compulsory screening of homosexuals, immigrants and drug addicts and the forced internment of those found to be positive. In 1985 the British government introduced special legislation to allow the compulsory detention of Aids patients in hospital—a world first in repressive legislation against Aids sufferers. Proposals to deprive Aids sufferers of employment rights and introduce quarantine regulations (Proposition 64) were defeated last year in California.

It is widely acknowledged that contact-tracing by special clinics helped to curb the spread of VD even before the discovery of antibiotics. But when naming somebody as a homosexual can lead to social disaster, contact-tracing is not likely to make much headway in the prevention of Aids today.

One illustration of this problem is the way that gay men have continued to donate blood lest a refusal to do so identify them as homosexual to family and friends. The North London Blood Transfusion Centre recently reported how, when a bisexual man came with his wife and a homosexual man came with his mother, both women were unaware of the men's homosexual activities (*Guardian,* 6 February 1987). The introduction of a special box on the blood donation form, however, allowed the men confidentially to notify the staff. They could thus donate blood without giving things away to their relatives; meanwhile their blood could be discarded.

For as long as homosexuality remains an underground activity in Britain, it will be impossible to prevent Aids spreading among gay men.

No safety

There is no such thing as safe sex if you have sex with other people. Masturbation is the only truly safe form of sex, now that modern medicine has conclusively discounted old myths about it causing blindness. Celibacy is the only lifestyle that can promise to deliver you from all fear of Aids.

Sex between human beings has always been a risky business.

Heterosexual sex often carries the risk of pregnancy, itself a life-threatening experience for a woman until recent years. Heterosexual sex also carries the risk for both partners of a wide range of sexually transmissible diseases, most of them extremely nasty. Sex between gay men can transmit all the same diseases, and, with anal intercourse, quite a few more. Even lesbian sex, although safer, can transmit venereal diseases.

Most people take a fairly pragmatic view of the dangers of sex. After all, life itself is dangerous. It is not safe to breathe the air in most Western cities, and after Chernobyl you can't even rely on the rainwater. Living in cities is dangerous, driving a car is very dangerous, being a passenger is even more dangerous, being at work is extremely dangerous. For any individual it makes sense to take appropriate precautions against the dangers in life. It makes sense to cross at a Zebra crossing, wear a seatbelt, wash your hands after going to the toilet...and to use a condom if you have sex with someone you don't know very well. We didn't need the government to spend £20m to tell us this.

For an individual it makes sense to take appropriate safety precautions in every area of life. But the Aids epidemic is a problem for society as a whole; it cannot be dealt with on an individual basis.

From the point of view of the individual the safe sex campaign is at worst alarmist, at best banal. From the point of view of society as a whole the campaign provides no answer to the real, if limited, problem of Aids. History shows that repression and exhortation are ineffective methods of changing public behaviour, especially in the sphere of sex.

A rational response to the Aids epidemic would set about getting rid of all forms of discrimination against homosexuals and ensure adequate resources for research into a cure and vaccine for HIV infection and for all aspects of the care of Aids sufferers. The government's safe sex campaign puts the bulk of its resources into promoting a scare campaign that has the effect of reinforcing the repression of homosexuals, while providing minimal funds for practical measures against Aids.

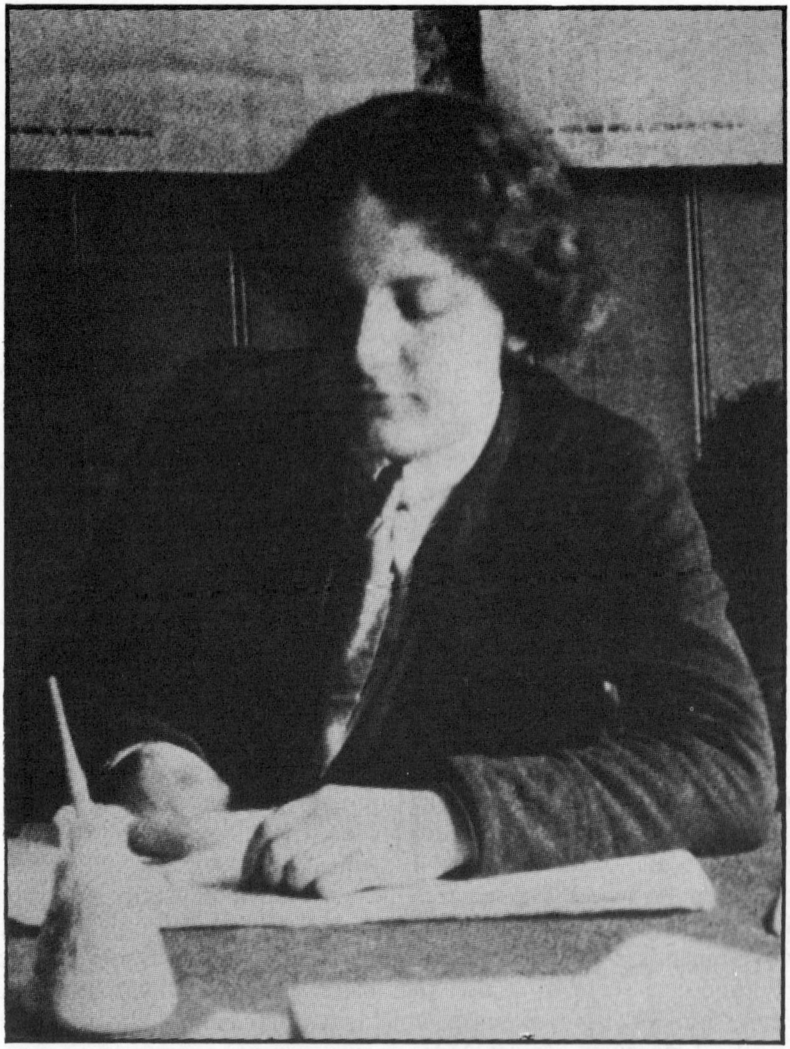

Christabel Pankhurst: the suffragettes' support for the social purity movement drew them into line with the establishment (see page 45)

5. The new moralism

The safe sex campaign has forged a wide consensus of support, stretching from right-wing religious fundamentalists to the gay movement. The medical establishment has provided a scientific rationale for this convergence around a campaign to change the moral and sexual behaviour of society.

In the USA, Jerry Falwell, one of the leaders of the right-wing evangelical revival, has declared that 'Aids is the wrath of God upon homosexuals'. In Britain, James Anderton, chief constable of Manchester and born-again Christian, has preached a similar theme: 'I ask why homosexuals freely engage in sodomy—let's be blunt about it—and other obnoxious practices, knowing the dangers involved.' Referring to modern society as 'a swirling human cesspit', Anderton described Aids as 'a self-inflicted scourge' and appealed for tougher measures against homosexuals.

The churches have taken advantage of the Aids panic to reaffirm traditional condemnations of homosexuality and to assert the virtues of chastity and monogamy. On behalf of the Catholic Church, Cardinal Ratzinger, the Pope's all-purpose hatchetman, has proclaimed homosexuality an abomination, recalling the destruction of the biblical cities of Sodom and Gomorrah as a punishment for their licentious behaviour (see *The Tablet,* 8 November 1986). Closer to home, Cardinal Basil Hume has insisted that 'people must cut out sexual permissiveness and promiscuity if the Aids epidemic is to be contained' (*Daily Telegraph,* 2 December 1986). He decreed that 'the sexual expression of love' should be 'reserved to marriage'.

Characteristically, the Church of England has taken a more pragmatic approach. John Hapgood, Bishop of York, has criticised the fundamentalist Anderton for stirring up prejudice against Aids sufferers on the grounds that this would 'drive them underground', which would 'prove dangerous' (*Guardian,* 7 January 1987). However, he too emphasises that the central lesson of Aids is the 'need to recover wise social taboos'. He calls for homosexuals and others to recognise 'a profound need for a change in their lifestyles' towards traditional Christian lines.

The common theme of the churches and the fundamentalist right is that Aids is the ultimate reward for promiscuity and permissiveness. The moral majority was on the march, calling for curbs on homosexuality, pornography, contraception and abortion and for a return to conventional family values, long before Aids struck. The Aids epidemic has given the promoters of the new conservatism a tremendous boost. It has allowed them to portray the seventies as the decade that began with the pill, but 'ended with Aids'. The fears aroused by the Aids panic provide a receptive audience for sermons on the virtues of sexual restraint and the sanctity of marriage.

In Britain, the government has carefully kept its distance from the overtly anti-gay rhetoric of the religious right. Home secretary Douglas Hurd described Anderton's outburst of bigotry as 'unhelpful'. Health minister Norman Fowler declared that demands from Staffordshire county councillor Bill Brownhill for the gassing of homosexuals were 'unacceptable'.

The government's own propaganda has been presented in scrupulously neutral terms, eschewing any tone of condemnation or moralism. However, as Fowler explained at the launch of the government's safe sex campaign, this is more a division of labour than a fundamental difference of outlook. He emphasised that 'the government's aim of teaching prudence is complementary to the teachings of the church and other religious leaders.' The government is happy for the professional moralists to take the lead in condemning homosexuality and promiscuity, while it issues sober public health propaganda which carries the same basic message in a more discreet manner.

The medical role

In both Britain and the USA the medical profession has played a pivotal role in the Aids panic. Gay doctors have helped to found and staff Aids organisations. In Britain the Gay Medical Association has worked closely with the Terrence Higgins Trust: the trust's early leaflets all carried the legend 'compiled with the help and advice of doctors'.

Traditional medical prejudices have not disappeared overnight. The *Southern Medical Journal* in the USA still insists that 'homosexuality is a pathologic condition.' Dr John Dawson, head of the British Medical Association's professional division, caused a furore in January when he advised anybody who had had more than one sexual partner in the past four years not to donate blood. The staff of the national blood transfusion service, which relies on donations from young people, were horrified at the prospect of a dramatic fall in supplies. Within days the BMA was forced to eat Dawson's words. However, the medical establishment in general has welcomed the opportunities provided by the Aids panic.

For doctors, anything which puts the disease in the headlines must be good news. The Aids panic has created pressures for funding for research projects, special wards and hospital posts as well as for a host of specialist counsellors and advisers. With a keen eye for a potential medical growth area, teaching hospitals such as St Mary's and the Middlesex in London have been quick to come up with schemes which attract publicity, and, with publicity, money. At a time of retrenchment in health service spending, especially in inner London, this is the only way to keep academic medicine and hospital facilities in business.

'Patients are being turned away, wait for long periods, or are given more rapid care than is desirable' declared two professors and a dean from the Middlesex hospital in a letter to the health minister appealing for more funds for Aids patients. But this description applies to every area of care under the national health service, from GP surgeries to heart transplant units. It is true that the resources allocated to Aids are inadequate. But how much more inadequate are the resources provided for public health problems much bigger than Aids, such as Britain's scandalous levels of perinatal mortality, or its limited kidney transplant and dialysis programmes?

Last year, Dr Kenneth Jones, district medical officer for North Lincolnshire, wrote an extensive account of his work in setting up 'a practical information network' on Aids in his local area (see *Health Trends,* August 1986). This involved setting up 'a multi-disciplinary

Aids advisory group' of consultants, nursing officers and administrators; issuing comprehensive guidelines on the protection of staff; holding seminars for education authorities, GPs, social service personnel, the police and undertakers; and producing information packs for the media and the general public. At the close of his article, Dr Jones makes a remarkable admission: 'The incidence of Aids infection in North Lincolnshire is low—there have not been any cases recorded.' If this is so, the incidence of Aids is not low, it is zero—Aids is simply a non-problem in North Lincolnshire. Dr Jones boldly concedes that 'In these circumstances it may seem the efforts have been excessive,' but pleads that it is as well to be prepared. While the medical authorities go to such absurd lengths to cope with non-existent diseases, hundreds of real health problems are neglected.

The case of North Lincolnshire is an extreme example, but the same approach to Aids is widespread. In East London, for example, where there are a few Aids cases, the authorities have appointed three specialist Aids officers. Meanwhile, tuberculosis and other diseases of poverty run rampant without any special public health effort to stop them.

Medical enthusiasm for Aids is not merely a cynical drive to win more resources for a disease in vogue. It also arises from the potential provided by Aids for doctors to extend their function as guardians of public morality. The fact that medical attempts to conquer Aids are so ineffectual has given a particular impetus for doctors to take to the television studios to pontificate on sexual behaviour in society. It has also led to a 're-medicalisation' of homosexuality, after a decade in which gay men and lesbians defied the pseudo-scientific theories with which generations of medical experts have tried to rationalise prevailing prejudices.

Social purity revisited

There is a striking parallel between today's safe sex campaign and the 'social purity' movement against venereal diseases in the early years of this century. The social purity campaign brought together right-wing moralists, the leading suffragette organisations and prominent members of the medical profession in calling for a change in sexual behaviour as the only way to stop the spread of gonorrhoea and syphilis. According to one historian of the movement, social purity suffragettes 'wanted the state to act in its public health capacity as a moralising agency—to discourage promiscuity and encourage responsible sexual relations through moral education' (Lucy Bland,

'Cleansing the Portals of Life: The Venereal Disease Campaign in the Early Twentieth Century', in Mary Langan and Bill Schwartz, editors, *Crises in the British State, 1880-1920,* 1985).

In the years around the First World War the suffragette movement was virtually taken over by the social purity campaign and its agitation against prostitution and male hypocrisy. Writing in 1908, Louisa Martindale, herself a doctor and a leading campaigner for women's rights, insisted that the fight for women's suffrage was 'a moral movement'. It included in its aims 'a desire to purify, by means of good laws, the social life of the people'. In 1910 suffragettes, clerics, doctors and radical politicians came together in the National Council for Public Morals. Under the title of the Association for Moral and Social Hygiene, a similar coalition led a campaign for safe sex through the war and into the twenties.

The social purity campaigners identified sexual licence as a threat to the stability of the family, the race, the nation and the Empire. In 1913, in her book *The Great Scourge and How to End It,* Christabel Pankhurst argued that venereal diseases were 'the great cause of physical, mental and moral degeneracy and of race suicide'. She coined the catchy slogan 'Votes for women, chastity for men.' Not all feminists went along with the social purity movement. The novelist Rebecca West dismissed Pankhurst's remarks as 'utterly valueless and likely to discredit the cause in which we believe'. She observed that 'this scolding attitude...is also a positive incentive to keep these diseases the secret spreading thing they are ' (quoted in Bland). Yet, while West fought for sexual freedom for both women and men, most of the movement followed Pankhurst into the grip of reaction.

Germ fever

In the USA in the same period, doctors helped to promote a public health panic which had a lasting effect on women's position in society. The 'germ theory' provoked a wave of public anxiety about the dangers of 'contagion' from ill-defined microscopic organisms (see Barbara Ehrenreich and Deirdre English, *For Her Own Good: 150 Years of the Experts' Advice to Women,* 1979). Popular magazine titles from the period 1900 to 1904 convey the atmosphere: 'Books Spread Contagion', 'Contagion by Telephone', 'Infection and Postage Stamps,' 'Disease from Public Laundries', 'Menace of the Barber Shop'.

Medical science gave full backing to the drive to turn women into professional housekeepers, trained in the subtleties of the newly invented discipline of 'domestic science'. The American Medical

Association regarded the housewife as the front line in the battle against the germs:

> 'Medical men who know the value of a trained nurse can readily appreciate the value of a training which will not only make American wives prudent, economic and thrifty, but which will establish a sanitary regime in every room in the home as well as in the kitchen and dining room.'(quoted in Ehrenreich and English)

Cleaning became a sanitary crusade; keeping a hygienic household was now a moral responsibility. Advertisements for soap and detergents played on maternal fears of contagion and guilt over the slightest neglect of cleanliness.

The domestic science movement rapidly incorporated the bulk of the American women's movement. The result of this convergence of medical authority with feminist zeal was to tie women to a new range of domestic tasks at the very time when the growing availability of consumer durables had reduced the burden of housework. The germ theory panic showed how fears of contagion could be manipulated to help preserve the status quo.

The history of the social purity and domestic science campaigns has made the women's movement sceptical about taking doctors' orders unquestioningly. Unfortunately the role of the medical profession in the Aids panic has yet to provoke a similar scepticism from the gay movement.

6. Aids and the gay movement

Ten years ago any suggestion of the possibility of a convergence between the gay movement and the religious right would have been dismissed as a bizarre joke. Yet, under the banner of safe sex, these unexpected bedfellows have come together. How did this happen?

Before the seventies there was little gay movement. Leadership fell to discreet and moderate bodies devoted to lobbying for legislative reforms. These bodies were overwhelmingly middle class and respectable, acting partly as contact organisations for isolated homosexuals and as reformist pressure groups. Typical were the Mattachine Society in the USA, and the Homosexual Law Reform Society and Campaign for Homosexual Equality in Britain. While lesbians were sometimes included in these bodies, they also set up their own organisations of a similar type (see John D'Emilio, *Sexual Politics, Sexual Communities: The Making of a Homosexual Minority in the United States, 1940-1970,* 1983; and Jeffrey Weeks, *Coming Out: Homosexual Politics in Britain, from the Nineteenth Century to the Present,* 1977).

Given the enormous institutionalised prejudice, discrimination and brutality endured by homosexuals—and the failure of the labour movement and left to defend their rights—the overwhelmingly defensive and inward-looking character of homosexual organisation was to be expected. As a wider political force, gay organisation only really took off in the seventies.

The transformation of a movement

In the seventies there was a wave of homosexual activity as middle class youth took up Vietnam, student power, black power, women's rights and trade union militancy. In the USA, the Stonewall riot in New York in 1969, when gays fought back against police harassment of gay bars, provided a focus for gay radicalisation; so did the campaign for political representation around Harvey Milk in San Francisco in the early seventies. In Britain the Gay Liberation Front took to the streets, challenging the state, the left and the established gay organisations with equal vigour and enthusiasm.

In their heyday the gay movements of the seventies sought individual emancipation through a cathartic and collective defiance of established sexual mores. 'Queers' and 'lezzies' redefined themselves proudly as gay men and lesbians; 'coming out' became the crucial first step to liberation. This is how Jeffrey Weeks summed up the basic concepts of the Gay Liberation Front:

> 'First the idea of 'coming out', of being open about one's homosexuality, of rejecting the shame and guilt and the enforced 'double life', of asserting 'gay pride' and 'gay anger' around the cry, 'Out of the closets, into the streets.' Secondly the idea of 'coming together', of solidarity and strength coming through collective endeavour, and of mass confrontation of oppression. And thirdly, and centrally, the identification of the roots of oppression in the concept of sexism, and of exploring means to extirpate it.' (*Coming Out,* p191)

However, the gay movement's hopes of a 'mass confrontation of oppression' have been dashed. Something was missing from even the most radical perspectives of the Gay Liberation Front. The gay movement of the early seventies failed to realise that the oppression of homosexuals results not merely from the anti-gay attitudes of straight society, or even from the way in which these values have become internalised by most homosexuals. The oppression of homosexuality is bound to be institutionalised in a society in which the family is fundamental to reproducing the working class and keeping it under control.

The impact of the world recession in the mid-seventies turned the tide against all radical movements. Growing social conflict and political instability made it more important than ever for the authorities to bolster up the family and family values as a source of authority and discipline in society. Pressures to curb departures from conventional sexual behaviour and the norms of family life intensified. On its own, the gay movement lacked the strength to challenge modern society at its foundations and it rapidly crumbled in the attempt.

The gay movement fragmented. Gay men and lesbians, reformists and revolutionaries, gay theatre groups and gay rock bands, Christian, Jewish and infidel homosexuals all went their separate ways. In his extensive survey of the impact of Aids on the US gay scene, Denis Altman comments that while the gay scene expanded, by the late seventies it had 'lost any claim to ideological coherence' (*Aids and the New Puritanism,* 1986). By 1980 Ronald Reagan had substantial gay support in his election campaign (he chose, however, to keep quiet about it).

The main beneficiaries of the greater space created for homosexuals in Western cities by the radical movement of the seventies were the gay entrepreneurs. The proprietors of bathhouses, gay clubs and bars, gay newspapers and magazines flourished. While radical gay politics languished, the gay millionaire made his appearance.

The assassination of Harvey Milk by Dan White, his homophobic rival in the San Francisco municipal politics of 1978, signalled the changing climate. White was acquitted on the grounds of diminished responsibility resulting from depression induced by eating junk food. San Francisco gays rioted in outrage but the gay community was already on the defensive. The moral majority was campaigning for restrictions on homosexuality—itself still outlawed in half the states of the Union—in the 1980 presidential elections, before anybody had heard of Aids. Thus when Aids arrived the gay scene in the USA was already retreating in disarray before the renewed moral offensive.

In Britain, things were even worse. Here the gay movement never reached the scale of that in the USA, with its vast gay pride marches and flourishing cultural life, particularly in San Francisco and New York. It emerged later and proved less durable. The 1983 wrangle between radicals and entrepreneurs for the control of *Gay News,* Britain's most successful gay newspaper, symbolised the strife in the movement. Significantly, the entrepreneurs, personified by editor/proprietor Denis Lemon, came out on top. However, a distinctive feature of the demise of gay radicalism in Britain was the role played by the Labour Party, and in particular by left-wing Labour councils.

Ken Livingstone took over the running of the Greater London Council in 1981; left-wing leaderships were subsequently elected in a number of inner-London boroughs and provincial cities. These radical Labour councils fostered close links between radical movements and the local government machine. During the years of Labour government in the late seventies the traditional left had lost direction and influence, a plight which also afflicted the women's movement, many black radicals—and the gay movement.

The leading members of the established groupings of the oppressed were generally closely associated with the traditional left and the Labour Party, even though the official labour movement at best gave them only token support. In the harsher climate of Thatcher's Britain in the early eighties, they sought refuge under the wing of Labour councils. It was a move for which they were to pay a heavy price.

Left-wing Labour councils provided jobs for a whole generation of radical activists, plus resources for special committees for women, blacks and gay rights. These committees sponsored 'anti-racist years' and promoted 'positive images' of the oppressed through library displays and school textbooks. Yet the councils did little to challenge the institutionalised discrimination against women and minorities in British society. Indeed, as major employers and providers of state services, the councils actively carried out such discrimination. For cxample, the GLC never provided adequate nursery facilities for its own employees, nor did it alter the ghettoisation of black people below the stairs in its own offices, or in the worst housing estates it handed over to other authorities to manage.

In return for fat salaries and token campaigns, the radicals of the seventies accepted the reduced horizons dictated by their Labour paymasters. The gay radicals too were housetrained in Labour's quangos. In return for a few grants for lesbian and gay centres and phone lines, they put off to the future the struggle against the criminalisation of homosexuality and the brutalisation of homosexuals. The Labour Party conference passed bland resolutions of support for gay rights, while it continued to provide a platform for delegates to express anti-gay prejudices. The quangoisation of the gay movement had the effect of softening it up before the Aids panic struck.

The Aids revival

Over the past three years a moribund gay movement in both the USA and in Britain has become rejuvenated and reorganised around the issue of Aids. The New York Gay Men's Health Crisis, the San Francisco Aids Foundation, the Shanti Project, the Terrence Higgins Trust—these have become the gay movement's most prominent representative organisations.

The Aids organisations have more in common with the reformist committees of the fifties than with the radical gay movements of more recent years. In the USA they are massive fund-raising charities, concerned with everything from research, through counselling, to hospital and community-based care and support. They are also centrally involved in promoting safe sex and in acting as a pressure group on federal, state and municipal government. In Britain, the Terrence Higgins Trust carries out similar work on a much smaller scale.

In his account of Aids in the USA, Denis Altman comments: 'The most obvious impact of Aids has been to produce a new professional leadership in the gay movement, one whose legitimacy is based on expertise rather than on either movement experience or popular representation' (*Aids and the New Puritanism*). He adds that 'even under the Reagan administration, Aids has produced more contact between the gay movement and federal officials than ever before.' He also notes that 'the other side to these developments is that the pressures to respond to the constant crises posed by Aids divert attention from other matters of concern to the gay movement, such as discrimination in general, violence, immigration and even other health issues.'

If gay liberation brought gays out of the closet like never before, the reorganisation of the gay movement around Aids has made the movement's leadership more a part of the system and less in touch than ever with the real problems of gay oppression.

The safe sex campaign has brought the gay movement full circle. From being in the vanguard of calls for sexual experimentation, it has come round to making vigorous statements demanding restraint and responsibility. It has become commonplace for erstwhile gay radicals to confess their feelings of guilt at their past advocacy of libertine attitudes. Altman concludes with a statement of personal contrition:

> 'It is difficult in view of the restrictions imposed by Aids to escape the feeling that those of us who argued for liberating sex in the sixties and seventies were wrong.'

He notes with approval the fact that Aids 'has led gay men to go beyond a preoccupation with sex and partying to a new evaluation of community and family'. For all its repudiations of the religious right, the gay movement appears to have accepted its basic message that homosexual promiscuity is responsible for the spread of Aids and that gays must now adopt a life of caution.

Transcendental labourism

One of the leading safe sex campaigners in Britain is Peter Tatchell, a Labour Party activist who was disowned by his party leadership and viciously gay-baited in the press when he stood as a parliamentary candidate in the Bermondsey by-election in 1983. Tatchell's book *Aids: A Guide to Survival* (1986) provides a detailed account of safe sex techniques, claiming that 'on this issue at least the gay and lesbian communities have asserted a moral leadership which has been significantly lacking from other quarters in society.' Tatchell goes so far as to criticise the churches for neglecting their responsibilities for giving 'moral leadership' in the sphere of sexual behaviour.

Tatchell recognises the irony of his position as a gay activist preaching a similar message to that of the moral majority:

> 'To some the restrictiveness of safe sex unhappily echoes the homophobia and puritanism of the new right: witness the Conservative government's fierce defence of 'family life' and its call for a return to 'Victorian values'! Yet in the absence of a medical cure for Aids, it is hard to see how either gay people or heterosexuals have any real alternative.'

Tatchell goes on in increasingly portentous terms, proclaiming that our options are limited and that we must choose between 'survival or suicide'.

These 'alternatives' are entirely bogus. Because 680 people in Britain, 97 per cent of them male homosexuals, haemophiliacs, drug abusers or their babies, have contracted a sexually transmissible disease, the whole population should resort to masturbation, monogamy or the use of condoms? How ridiculous! Since there is as yet no medical cure for Aids, the first priority should be to find one, not to try to use the disease to scare the whole nation into a return to Victorian values. Not only is this wholly undesirable: it is also no answer to the problem of Aids.

Until a cure for Aids is found, the only alternative is to fight to remove the stigmatisation of homosexuality that is the main factor in creating the conditions in which HIV spreads. Unfortunately this is the very task that has been abandoned by the gay movement in its headlong rush to promote safe sex.

Tatchell's book reveals one of the most disturbing features of the gay movement's response to Aids—a profound fatalism that leads to a resort to mysticism and other flights from reality. One illustration of this is the way in which the author almost rejoices in the impact of the safe sex campaign on the gay scene:

'Increasingly gay men are dating before sex and getting into deeper, long-term love affairs. Greater value is being placed on caring, supportive friendships. Responsibility is becoming the catchword in personal relationships and, in echoes of the fifties, romance is back in fashion.'

The other 'echo of the fifties'—as Tatchell himself admits—is that queer-bashing is back in fashion. In the real world, where the Aids panic has given a new ferocity to anti-gay prejudice, the prospects of stable relationships for the vast majority of gay men are gloomier than ever. For homosexuals in a hostile world, 'romance' is more and more illusory.

Tatchell's guide to fighting Aids with 'meditation, mental imagery and positive mental reinforcement' recalls the religious revivals that followed the plague epidemics of the Middle Ages. It is difficult to see how standing in front of a mirror reiterating the will to get well (the basic technique of mental imagery) can have much effect in rallying a disintegrating immune system. Nor is it easy to imagine the advance of pneumocystis carinii pneumonia or Kaposi's sarcoma being slowed by Aids patients recalling the heroic exploits of Douglas Bader or Francis Chichester, part of the mental reinforcement programme recommended by Tatchell. When the author concludes on different methods of reducing stress, he suggests: 'Laughter is probably the best medicine of all.' The most worrying thing is that he isn't joking.

Altman quotes a letter from an Aids patient to a gay paper in the USA which highlights a prevalent theme in the gay movement's response to Aids:

'I would rather live one year with this disease than 50 years of my previous lifestyle. I have never been so loved or closer to my purpose in life.'

This may be a tribute to the quality of care that the American gay movement has mobilised for those suffering from Aids. But it is also a grim testimony to the quality of life endured by most gays in modern society—that dying of Aids is preferable to living as a homosexual. How tragic that, while working overtime to ensure that its members die peacefully, the gay movement has given up the fight for day-to-day freedom and dignity. Indeed by endorsing the safe sex campaign, it has given its approval to the continuing suppression of gay rights.

The Terrence Higgins Trust, the main voluntary body concerned with Aids in Britain, is not as moralistic as Tatchell. Its propaganda, like that of the government, is written in a more matter-of-fact tone, with a greater air of scientific authority. However, the trust's leaflets have made a significant contribution to the Aids panic.

The Terrence Higgins Trust has gone to great lengths to classify every conceivable form of sexual activity into one of five risk categories (none, low, medium, higher and highest). While it acknowledges that it is 'exceptionally rare' for people outside the high-risk categories to become infected with the Aids virus, its guidelines are offered for the entire population. A rational approach to the Aids problem would distinguish between those in the high-risk categories, for whom special precautions may be necessary, and the vast majority of the population, who can be reassured that they have little to fear from Aids.

Issuing detailed safe sex guidelines to the whole nation can only arouse unnecessary fears and anxieties. Even for those in the high-risk groups a much simpler classification is justified given the present state of scientific knowledge. This would designate receptive anal intercourse and possibly vaginal intercourse with anybody likely to be HIV-positive as relatively risky and everything else as relatively safe. However, the more detailed the discussion of different sexual activities, the more the preoccupation with Aids is encouraged—and this is exactly what is required for the spread of a moral panic.

The very banality of some of the advice issued by the Terrence Higgins Trust contributes to the general hysteria. Here is the trust's list of suggestions for maintaining hygiene in a household where somebody is suffering from HIV infection:

* make sure meat is properly defrosted and cooked through
* wash up in water and detergents hot enough to need gloves
* use different cleaning and washing cloths for kitchen and bathroom
* wear gloves for gardening
* wash hands after handling pets or pet litter trays.

There are many more novel household tips: 'Any cuts or grazes you have should be covered over by a waterproof dressing until a scab has formed.' The trust is also ready with advice for women: 'Used sanitary towels and tampons', it says, 'should be flushed down the toilet, or put in a sealed plastic bag.' What a good idea!

Are these measures really vital in the fight against Aids? Or do they simply indicate a fastidious trend in the gay movement? Or is it simply that the Terrence Higgins Trust likes issuing lists of instructions to the public?

Like naughty boys who have been made into school prefects, the gay radicals of the past now promote sexual restraint with greater zeal than they ever did the cause of sexual liberation. Whereas in the seventies their activities faced censorship and repression, they now find themselves receiving open endorsement from the highest level of state. The government recommended the Terrence Higgins Trust phone line to 23 million households in its special Aids leaflet, though there was some doubt whether the organisation's limited phone lines could cope if everybody actually rang for safe sex advice.

For the leading activists in the Aids movement, the government's backing for safe sex is an indication that the gay movement has come of age as a political force. In fact, however, it shows that the gay movement has been destroyed as a progressive force. Even for professional Aids campaigners, the honeymoon of establishment approval cannot last. Once the safe sex campaign has run its course and the backlash against homosexuality gathers momentum, the respectable leaders of the gay community too will suffer the consequences.

Dodging the issue

'Too little, too late'—this was the universal response of the gay movement and the left to the government's campaign against Aids. Scarcely anybody objected to the central thrust of the campaign—the urgent need for everybody to practise safe sex as the only way of halting the spread of the Aids virus. Instead there was a chorus of criticism of the government's delay in launching the publicity campaign and its failure to put adequate resources into it. Radical papers echoed calls from doctors and politicians for more explicit commercials, and demanded more emphasis on the virtues of condoms and spermicides.

The defect of the radical response to Aids is that it unquestioningly accepts the official views that Aids is a major threat to public health and that the call for safe sex is a rational response. Indeed, the left often exaggerates the danger even more than the authorities, to justify its condemnations of the government's alleged incompetence and its own emphasis on the practicalities of safe sex.

For example, this is how one socialist newspaper responded to the launch of the government campaign last November:

> 'The only short-term way of slowing the spread of the disease is through safe sex. This means making sure that everyone knows what precautions they can take. But unless the campaign is uncompromisingly open and explicit, it will be counter-productive. The government's campaign must openly say that everyone should use condoms.' (*Socialist Worker*, 22 November)

Within weeks the government's leaflet was openly saying just that in 23 million households. While the left joined in the national condom promotion drive (one paper suggested that the London Rubber Company should become a prime target for social ownership under a future Labour government), it overlooked the artificial and irrational character of the whole Aids panic. It has also evaded the political problem that Aids has pushed to the centre of attention—the issue of lesbian and gay rights.

In their defensive response to Aids, the gay movement and the left have endorsed the government scare about HIV spreading among heterosexuals. Writing in *Marxism Today* in January, Jeffrey Weeks, the historian of gay politics in Britain, took exception to the label 'gay plague', partly because it 'encourages those who do not see themselves as gay to believe that they will not get it'. From the Terrence Higgins Trust to the Communist Party, everybody is at pains to play up the risk of Aids to heterosexuals.

The left's focus on the heterosexual spread of Aids appears to arise from a concern to take the heat generated by the Aids panic off the gay community. In practice it merely assists the government in spreading the Aids panic among heterosexuals. In fact, as we have seen, heterosexuals are in very little danger of contracting Aids. Homosexual men, however, are not only the main high-risk group, but are also the main victims of the panic. Scaring straights is no way to protect gays from the anti-homosexual backlash generated around the fear of HIV contagion.

Some radical commentators on Aids have drawn attention to other high-risk categories apart from gay men. But this simply offers additional targets for prejudice and repression. The high incidence of the disease in Africa has already been used to justify even tighter immigration regulations and to legitimise wider hatred of black immigrants. Bisexuals have been blamed for acting as a bridge between the gay scene and straight society. Some radical gays have pursued the safe sex line to the conclusion that everybody should adopt an exclusively heterosexual or exclusively homosexual orientation.

The radical response to the Aids scare reaches its most absurd in criticisms of top Tories for their failure to live up to the moral code which they seek to impose on the rest of society. The names of disgraced party officers Cecil Parkinson and Jeffrey Archer figure prominently in the left's attempts to outdo the right in its moralism and priggishness. What better demonstration of the success of their campaign could the Tories wish for, than to hear their own sermons echoed from the platforms of the left?

The slogan 'No socialism without lesbian and gay liberation' used to be widely heard in left-wing circles. The response of the official labour movement to the Aids scare should deepen the already widespread scepticism among gays about Labour's commitment to upholding the rights of homosexuals. When Aids was debated in parliament last November, Labour frontbench spokesman Michael Meacher stated that he thought that it was 'right that this should be treated as a national crisis and above party politics'. But Aids is not a 'national crisis'. It is a rare disease that is spreading among homosexuals because of their inferior and persecuted position in society. It is also being skilfully exploited to stir up fears and prejudices among the rest of society.

Nor is the Aids scare an issue on which a party that claims to represent the labour movement can refuse to take up a distinctive position. Aids is a challenge to the official labour movement to take a stand in repudiating the drive to restore Victorian values, and in defending the rights of lesbians and gays. Labour's refusal to take up this challenge is a measure of its irrelevance to the problems of homosexual oppression that have been intensified by the Aids panic.

7. Family values and lesbian and gay rights

It is astonishing that the Thatcher line on Aids is so widely taken at face value. But why should the Tories be concerned about a rare disease which virtually exclusively affects gay men and drug abusers? Over the past seven years, the Tory government has created suffering and misery on a scale that dwarfs the best efforts of the puny Aids virus. The Tories' corporate paymasters kill workers by the hundred every year without provoking a multi-million pound campaign of accident prevention. The Tories have cut back medical research, closed hospitals and dumped thousands of mentally ill and handicapped people back on their own families in 'the community'. Yet, all of a sudden, 'public health' has become a matter for cabinet-level discussion.

The truth is that the British government could not care less if thousands of gays and drug abusers died of Aids. It is not even much concerned about the danger of the spread of Aids to heterosexuals, knowing as it does that the risk is slight. No, the establishment has thrown its weight behind the Aids panic because it recognises how the virus can help it strengthen its faltering grip over society.

The value of the Aids panic for the establishment is that it provokes anxieties over the one human activity on which people are most vulnerable to feelings of insecurity, self-doubt and guilt. There is nothing like the fear of contracting a mysterious disease—one that is incurable and leads to a lingering, wasting death—to make even someone of limited sexual experience break out in a cold sweat. It may be irrational, but you can't help worrying....This is exactly the kind of preoccupation the government is trying to encourage.

So long as people are anxiously calculating their chances of being HIV-positive, thinking about how to practise sex safely and weighing up the pros and cons of condoms, their minds are kept safely away from unemployment, welfare cuts, declining wages, racism and war.

A Mori opinion poll conducted at the end of January, after the first stage of the government's Aids campaign, revealed that Aids had become the fifth most important issue for the British electorate. It was considered more important than education, pensions, defence and foreign policy. Significantly, the poll showed that women—who accounted for just 17 of the 610 cases of Aids up to the end of 1986—were even more worried than men: 14 per cent of women mentioned it as an issue compared with 9 per cent of men. The more isolated position of women in British society, at work and at home, makes them especially vulnerable to the fears and uncertainties generated by the Aids panic.

The Aids panic fits neatly into the government's wider drive to bolster conventional family values and proscribe all departures from these norms. The fear of picking up a lethal infection is a potent weapon with which to encourage young people to stay on the sexual straight and narrow. Hence a government which has previously sought to restrict sex education in schools is now keen to make sure that its Aids propaganda reaches down even to junior level. If there is little enough risk to adults from Aids, there is zero risk to school children. But never mind, the opportunity to hit impressionable minds with pro-family propaganda is too good to miss.

The message coming through the Aids panic is clear: promiscuity in general and homosexuality in particular are bad—restraint and marriage are good.

The Tories and the family

The family is a crucial institution in modern society. For the propertied classes, it provides a framework for passing on wealth and some accumulated wisdom of those experienced in running industry, the professions and government. More importantly, it provides the means by which workers are nurtured and cared for, from cradle to grave, and from generation to generation. The family also plays a key role in transmitting deference to authority and respect for law and order. Such values are essential to a society based on the subordination of the majority to a minority which monopolises economic and political power. Given the importance of the family for capitalists, they have always branded alternatives to family life as immoral or illegal, or both.

The climate of deepening economic and social crisis in modern Britain has a profound impact on family life. The strains resulting from mass unemployment and the slide of millions below the poverty line make it more and more difficult for many families to sustain the idealised image of family life constantly projected by the media. The result is record levels of divorce, family breakdown and single parenthood. Yet the more the recession destroys families, the more the politicians, the churches and the media are enlisted to proclaim the virtues of family life. That is why the promotion of the family has been the theme common to a series of moral panics under the Tories, from scares about surrogate motherhood to scandals about teenagers on the pill.

The first attempt to make the family an issue in British politics in recent times came from Labour leader James Callaghan in the 1979 election. Callaghan tried to distract attention from Labour's catastrophic record in government by projecting himself as the father of the nation and the personal representative of decent traditional values. Despite his parade of his wife, sons and daughters and grandchildren before the press, the nation was not impressed. It opted for the politician who has most consistently trumpeted personal responsibility and a sense of individual self-respect—Margaret Thatcher.

'Think about the family,' Thatcher told her ministers when she set up a special 'family policy group' shortly after her 1979 election victory. In September 1982 the group put forward a programme for dismantling state welfare provision and transferring responsibility for personal care on to the family. Its proposals included encouraging mothers to stay at home, encouraging schools with 'a clear moral base', extending home ownership, privatising sections of the social services, making parents responsible for anti-social behaviour on the part of their children, and promoting 'self-help' among the unemployed. Much of this programme has been introduced.

The Tories' promotion of the family has a number of purposes. First, the government aims to curb public spending by shifting the burden of welfare services on to the family. Cuts in spending on social security, health, education and local authority services have increased the load carried by the family. Looking after children, the sick, the old, the mentally ill and the disabled is increasingly the task of women in the home. 'Community care' in the family has saved the government billions.

Second, the Tories have tried to use the family as a source of discipline and control in times when violent repression and angry revolt are becoming increasingly commonplace. In 1985 Thatcher appealed for a strengthening of 'our traditional sources of discipline and authority'—the family, the church and the school—as part of her wider drive for law and order. The government has tried to bolster parental authority by giving parents a disciplinary role in Youth Training Schemes, and by refusing housing benefit to young people who leave home.

Third, family life emphasises individual preoccupations and undermines the possibility of collective resistance. To prove his fitness for high office, Neil Kinnock regularly reassures the media that he 'puts his family first'. This is an outlook that the establishment would like to see made universal; for as long as every man, woman and child is preoccupied with their own immediate relationships, and with their responsibility to maintain a certain standard of household, the system is safe. In any major strike, the media single out for praise the workers who put home and family first and go back to work.

For the working class, focusing on family life intensifies the isolation of individuals in society. In the narrow private sphere of personal relationships, all problems appear to be unique and individual. The solutions appear to lie in the phone helpline, the advice centre or even the police, rather than in collective organisation. A nation of families is a collection of isolated individuals, and that is how the Tories want to keep us.

Victims of family values

The main victims of the drive to restore family values are women. Women carry the burden of increased work in the home, acting as child-bearers and child-rearers, cooks, cleaners, nurses and providers of general household services. A heavier workload in the home makes it more difficult for women to get out to work and to participate in the wider life of society. Limited access to contraception and abortion reduces women's freedom to escape from the drudgery of child-bearing and child-rearing.

Women too carry the burden of the cares of holding the family together under the pressures of recession. These pressures often make them the victims of domestic violence and family breakdown. As heads of one-parent families, women are in an even more difficult position.

More and more, they are also the targets of public prejudice.

The reassertion of family life is also a threat to homosexuals. To foster a spirit of restraint and strengthen the marriage bond, the authorities may denounce heterosexual promiscuity. But Victorian values always allowed considerable flexibility is this area—so long as women were chaste, men could indulge themselves. Homosexuality, however, is a different matter: it must always be proscribed, because by its nature it threatens to undermine the family. This is why the attack on lesbian and gay rights has intensified in tandem with the wider revival of family values.

The oppression of homosexuals undermines the unity and cohesion of the whole working class. It creates suspicion and hostility among workers and helps the establishment impose its standards of conformity. It reinforces preoccupations about succeeding in heterosexual relationships and family life, and undermines workers' sense of collective organisation and collective activity. Hatred of homosexuals is invariably linked to chauvinist attitudes towards women.

When popular expressions of hostility towards homosexuals converge with the reactionary requirements of the state, moralism becomes a mighty weapon against the working class. The oppression of homosexuals and the cult of the family are features common to reactionary regimes from Hitler's Germany to Thatcher's Britain. This is why the defence of homosexuals is vital to asserting the unity of the working class.

For many, family relationships are a source of affection and intimacy. Fair enough, but that will not prevent the pressures of decaying capitalism from turning the family into a prison for many people, especially for women and homosexuals. We are not against the family as such, but we are resolutely opposed to its use as a device with which to suppress the working class and to restrict the rights of women, lesbians and gay men.

Aids and lesbian and gay rights

Many radical gays argue that Aids is such an immediate threat to life and health that safe sex is the only viable response in the short term. They regard the fight for lesbian and gay rights as something for the future, when the priority of survival is assured. But safe sex will not save lives as long as homosexuals remain oppressed. Indeed the anti-gay content of the safe sex campaign can only help to preserve the conditions of inferiority and vulnerability which leave gay men open to infection with HIV. Both in the long term and in the short term, the only way to save lives from Aids is by rejecting the panic that surrounds it and by fighting for the rights of lesbians and gay men.

The labour movement should fight for the removal of all legislation that discriminates against homosexuals. It should challenge every instance in which lesbians and gay men experience differential treatment because of their sexual orientation—whether this is at the hands of the courts, the police, employers, trade union officials, fellow workers, in the pub, in the street, anywhere. Instead of its traditional preoccupation with trying to radicalise the gay scene, the left should devote its energies to transforming the labour movement into an active force for lesbian and gay rights.

The safe sex campaign is a threat not only to homosexuals, but to the entire working class. By emphasising the virtues of restraint and monogamy, it promotes values that help to atomise the working class and undermine the will to take collective action. By defining the political problem of Aids as a personal matter of sexual preference and willingness to use condoms, the key questions at issue are obscured and avoided.

Combating the Aids scare means fighting for the equal treatment of homosexuals in society, and for the unity of the working class against divisive moralism and phoney public health propaganda.

Aids reading

Aids may be a new disease but the shelves of libraries and bookshops are already groaning under the weight of Aids literature. Here is a brief guide to a field in which books become out of date long before they are printed and articles in the medical and scientific journals provide the most useful source of up-to-date information.

Survey articles

ED ACHESON, 'Aids: A Challenge for the Public Health', ***The Lancet,*** 22 March 1986.

MADS MELBYE, 'The Natural History of Human T Lymphotropic Virus III Infection: The Cause of Aids', ***British Medical Journal,*** 4 January 1986.

ROBERT J BIGGAR, 'The Clinical Features of HIV Infection in Africa', ***British Medical Journal,*** 6 December 1986.

MERLE A SANDE, 'Transmission of Aids: The Case against Casual Contagion', ***New England Journal of Medicine,*** 6 February 1986.

NICOLAS WEBB, ***The Aids Virus: Forecasting Its Impact,*** Office of Health Economics, December 1986 (published as a pamphlet).

ROBERT C GALLO, 'The Aids Virus', ***Scientific American,*** January 1987.

Medical books

VICTOR GONG, ***Aids: A Comprehensive Guide,*** Cambridge, New York 1985. An American medical introduction written before the discovery of the Aids virus.

PETER EBBESON, ROBERT BIGGAR, MADS MELBYE, editors, ***Aids: A Basic Guide for Clinicians,*** Munksgaard, New York 1986. A more up-to-date survey by an international team of experts.

Popular introductions

JOHN GREEN and DAVID MILLER, ***Aids: The Story of a Disease,*** Grafton, London 1986. An account by two Aids counsellors from St Mary's hospital.

VG DANIELS, ***Aids: Questions and Answers,*** Cambridge Medical, London 1986. A brief and matter-of-fact British guide.

Scare propaganda

GRAHAM HANCOCK and ENVER CARIM, ***Aids: The Deadly Epidemic,*** Gollancz, London 1986. Low-life journalism devoted to promoting the panic.

DAVID BLACK, ***The Plague Years: A Chronicle of Aids,*** Pan, London 1986. The panic as presented in ***Rolling Stone*** magazine.

The radical response

DENIS ALTMAN, ***Aids and the New Puritanism,*** Pluto, London 1986. The definitive account of the impact of Aids on the gay scene in the USA by a well-known Australian writer on gay politics.

PETER TATCHELL, ***Aids: A Guide to Survival,*** GMP/Heretic, London 1986. The perspective of a prominent gay rights activist on the Labour left.

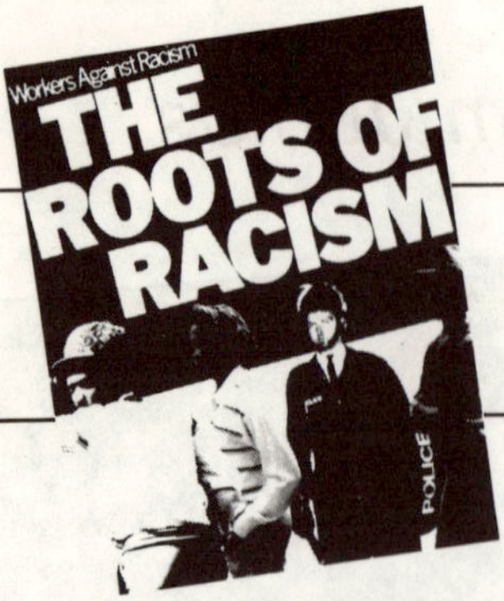

The Roots of Racism
Workers Against Racism
86 pages
£1.95 (plus 40p p&p)

The Soviet Union Demystified: A Materialist Analysis
Frank Füredi
304 pages
£5.95 paperback (plus 85p p&p)
£12.50 hardback (plus £1.20 p&p)

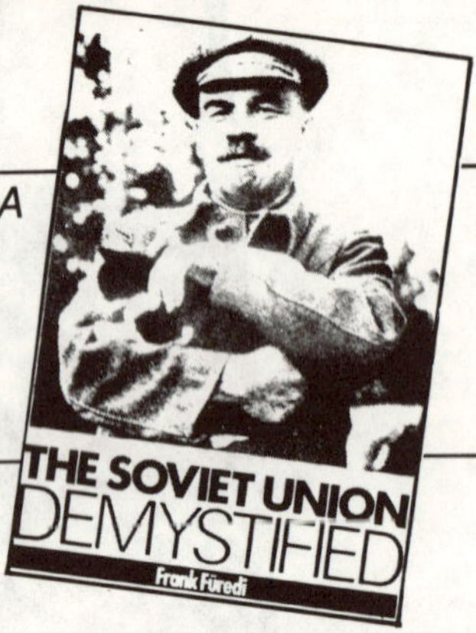

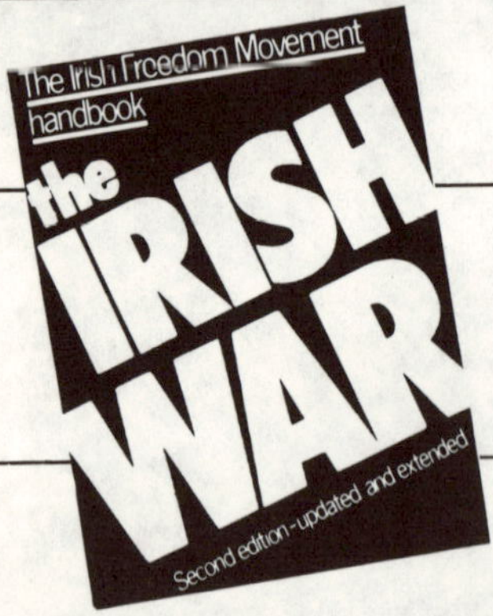

The Irish War:
The Irish Freedom Movement Handbook
252 pages
£2.95 (plus 60p p&p)

Taking Control: A Handbook for Trade Unionists
Mike Freeman
278 pages
£2.95 (plus 85p p&p)

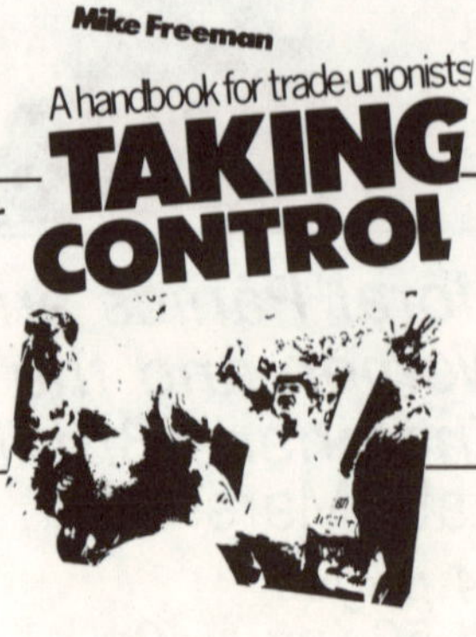

▶ Order from Junius Publications
BCM JPLtd
London WC1N 3XX
(01) 729 3771